MEDICINES for MAN
the development, regulation, and use of prescription drugs

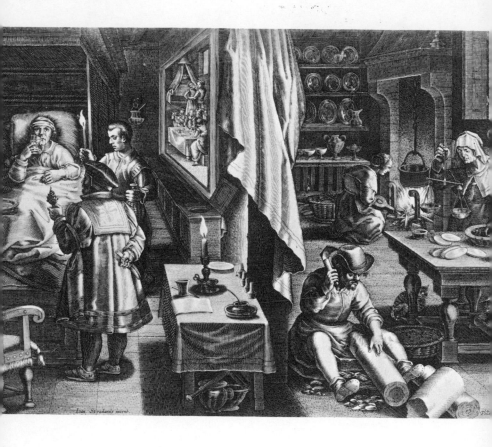

MEDICINES
for MAN

the development, regulation, and use of prescription drugs

HARRY F. DOWLING

1970 ALFRED · A · KNOPF *New York*

FRONTISPIECE: Guiac Being Prepared and
Administered for Syphilis *Engraving after J.
Van der Straet (Stradanus), published by Phillip
Galle in Nova Reperta, No. 6, Amsterdam, c.
1580. Reproduced from the collections of the
Library of Congress (LC-USZ62-26688)*

First Edition

Copyright © 1970 by Harry F. Dowling

All rights reserved under International and
Pan-American Copyright Conventions. Published
in the United States by Alfred A. Knopf, Inc.,
New York, and simultaneously in Canada by Random
House of Canada Limited, Toronto. Distributed
by Random House, Inc., New York.

Library of Congress Catalog Card Number: 73-98665

A portion of Chapter X was originally given in
a condensed version as a lecture, published and
reprinted by permission of The Johns Hopkins Press
from *Safeguarding the Public,* edited by Dr. John
Blake. Copyright © 1969 by The Johns Hopkins Press.

Manufactured in the United States of America

To My Three Sons,
FIL, LAINE, and JOHN,
each of whom contributed to
this book in his own way.

Preface

In the busy life of a physician-teacher, problems pop up one after the other. One gets into the habit of putting them aside in more or less orderly piles until he can give them the attention they deserve. In the course of caring for patients, teaching medical students and physicians, and carrying on research in infectious diseases for a third of a century, I encountered many problems that related to drugs. Service on various committees and boards, such as the Council on Drugs of the American Medical Association, the Revision Committee of the United States Pharmacopeia, and the Medical Advisory Board of the Food and Drug Administration brought answers to some questions and raised many more. Testifying before the subcommittees chaired by Congressman Blatnik and Senators Kefauver and Humphrey merely confirmed my impression that the dilemmas created by the conflicting interests of the several groups involved with drugs were not moving very rapidly toward solution.

At this point I had the good fortune to be appointed a Health Sciences Scholar of the National Library of Medicine. This enabled me to spend a sabbatical year at that institution rounding out my collection of facts and digging into the historical foundations of present-day practices in the discovery, development, regulation, and use of drugs.

In writing this book I have tried to give a balanced appraisal of the conflicting ideas and attitudes found at various points along the pathway from the conception to the consumption of drugs—balanced in time by a historical perspective, and balanced in philosophy by giving consideration to opposing opinions. Yet I have not hesitated at the end of each discussion of contrasting viewpoints to give my own, vulnerable though it may prove to be. For when a man asks for bread as food for action, who can hand him instead the stone of philosophy?

This book is for everyone who is concerned that he, his family, his friends, his patients, and people in general receive the best that this nation's technical skills can offer in the way of medicines to get them well or to keep them well, with a minimum of possibility for harm. It is written with sympathy for, and, I hope, with understanding of the problems of, those who are trying to bring more and better drugs to people, but with devotion to the welfare of the patients who are to receive the drugs as the ultimate criterion for action. As a physician, I have seen so many patients dramatically improved by drugs that I would want this to happen to everyone who can be helped, so many whose hopes were pinned on the outcome of a course of treatment that I would want to see such wishes fulfilled whenever possible. And I have sometimes seen suffering as a result of patients' receiving drugs that were improperly understood or ignorantly given; most of these tragedies I fervently hope can be prevented.

Many people have offered encouragement, ideas, and assistance of various kinds; these include administrators, physicians, pharmacists, biological and social scientists—in government, in the universities, in the drug industry, and elsewhere. My fellow committee members have informed and stimulated me and often set me straight both in and out of meetings.

Dr. Martin Cummings and his staff at the National Library of Medicine were most helpful in placing the facilities of that great library at my disposal. They consistently went far beyond the call of duty in responding to my requests. Particular thanks are due to Dr. John Blake and the other members of the Division of the History of Medicine. Dr. Blake not only gave frequent advice, but read the historical portions of the manuscript.

The Commissioners of Food and Drugs, Drs. James Goddard

and Herbert Ley; the Deputy Commissioner, Mr. Winton Rankin; the Director of the Division of Biologics Standards, Dr. Roderick Murray; the Directors of Revision of the United States Pharmacopeia, Drs. Lloyd Miller and William Heller; the Director of the Division of Scientific Activities and the Director of the Division of Drugs of the American Medical Association, Drs. Hugh Hussey and Thomas Hayes, and the Editor of the National Formulary, Dr. Edward Feldmann, arranged for me to obtain needed information about their organizations.

At various times during the past thirty years I have worked closely with a dozen pharmaceutical companies and have had occasional contacts with many more. These relationships were invaluable in giving me insight into the philosophy and workings of the modern pharmaceutical company. In preparation for writing this book, I consulted especially with Drs. Benjamin Carey, John Litchfield, W. G. Malcolm, William Parker, H. C. Peltier, James Ruegsegger, M. J. Schiffrin, Robert T. Stormont, William Sweeney, and Mr. Lyman Duncan and Mr. E. Claiborne Robins.

In London I was able to gain perspective by comparing the British and American systems of regulation of drugs through the kindness of Sir Derrick Dunlop and Dr. Dennis Cahal of the Committee on the Safety of Drugs of Great Britain, who gave generously of their time and arranged for me to talk with members of their staff. Among others in England who were helpful were Dr. D. R. Laurence of the University College Hospital, Dr. A. T. Mennie of Cyanamid, Ltd., Professor E. M. Titmuss of the London School of Economics and Political Science, and Mr. George Teeling-Smith of the Association of the British Pharmaceutical Industry. Visits with Drs. O. Wallen and Paul Blanc, present and former Chief Pharmacists of the World Health Organization, were also very productive.

I also profited from discussions with Dr. Paul Bunn of the State University of New York, Dr. Louis Lasagna of Johns

Hopkins University, Drs. Maxwell Finland, Osler Peterson, and David Rutstein of Harvard University, Dr. Leon Goldberg of Emory University, Professors S. J. Axelrod and Sylvester Berki of the University of Michigan, Henry Arthur, Bertrand Fox, and Curtis McLaughlin of Harvard University, Charlotte Muller of Columbia University, Alex Berman of the University of Texas, Dr. John Blair, Chief Economist, Senate Subcommittee on Antitrust and Monopoly, Dr. Morris Fishbein, formerly editor of the *Journal of the American Medical Association*, and Mr. Howard Binkley, Vice-President of the Pharmaceutical Manufacturers Association.

Special thanks are due to Professor James Harvey Young of Emory University, whose intimate knowledge of the history of food and drug legislation and regulation was invaluable to me, and Mr. Howard Wahrenbrock, former Solicitor of the Federal Power Commission, who straightened me out on many legal points and explained the procedures and idiosyncrasies of federal regulatory agencies.

Many persons, in addition to some of those mentioned, were kind enough to read portions of the manuscript, including: Drs. Wallace Janssen, Jean Lockhart, Robert McCleery, and Ralph Smith, Mr. William Goodrich and Mr. Julius Hauser of the Food and Drug Administration, Drs. Lester King and C. H. William Ruhe of the American Medical Association, Dr. Helen Potter of Purdue University, Dr. John Adriani of Tulane University, Professor Henry Steele of the University of Houston, and Drs. Nicholas Cotsonas, Clarence Gantt, Robert Herting, Richard Powers, and Alexander Schmidt, and Mr. Herbert Carlin of the University of Illinois.

Miss Irene Feldt read and re-read the manuscript and made many suggestions for improvement, and my secretary, Mrs. Joyce Fornek, supervised all stages of the enterprise from the preliminary accumulation of the data to the final preparation of the manuscript. I wish to thank, also, Miss Harlene Nystrom, Miss

Susan Baer, Mrs. Ruth Ackerman, Mr. Robert Adamczyk, Miss Natalie Brodzynsky, Miss Nancy Colburn, Miss Margarett Key, Miss Doris Mabins, and Miss Rhea Simons.

This work was supported in part by a Health Sciences Scholar Award of the National Library of Medicine, National Institutes of Health.

Contents

Abbreviations

ADE	*AMA Drug Evaluations*
AMA	American Medical Association
FDA	Food and Drug Administration
IND	Notice of Claimed Investigational Exemption for a New Drug
NDA	New Drug Application
NF	*The National Formulary*
NND	*New and Nonofficial Drugs*
NNR	*New and Nonofficial Remedies*
USP	*The United States Pharmacopeia*

MEDICINES for MAN
the development, regulation, and
use of prescription drugs

Some have cried one thing, and some another:
for the assembly was confused; and the more part
knew not wherefore they were come together.
—The Acts of the Apostles 19:32

The only way in which a human being can make
some approach to knowing the whole of a
subject, is by hearing what can be said about it
by persons of every variety of opinion. . . . No
wise man ever acquired his wisdom in any
way but this.
—JOHN STUART MILL, *On Liberty*

But every experiment is long and difficult, and
the laborers are few, and the number of facts
which we require to predict, enormous.
—HENRI POINCARÉ

Introduction

To one person the word "drugs" may mean a bottle of pink tablets in the medicine cabinet; to another, a group of addicts, drowsy from opiates or frenzied from cocaine; to a third, the injection he received before he was wheeled to the operating room. Actually, the word encompasses all of these and more. A drug may be defined as a substance used for the alleviation, improvement, cure, or prevention of a disease or its consequences. Taking drugs is a characteristically human trait, and everyone takes them sooner or later. Although drugs are also given to lower animals, those for humans are so much more numerous and create so many more problems that they alone will be considered in this book.

Medicines sold directly to the public are called "over-the-counter" drugs. They are well-known substances (or mixtures), whose effects have become familiar from decades or even centuries of usage. They are taken for minor symptoms, such as headaches, muscular aches, constipation, or nervous tension, and there are really only a few of them, although the number of remedies made from them and sold under various eye-catching trade names is legion.

New drugs, those used for serious illnesses or those having considerable potency for harm if misused, are called "prescription" drugs, because they can be dispensed only on order of a physician or a qualified practitioner in one of the other health professions. They have also been called, somewhat inaptly, "ethical" drugs, because it is considered unethical to advertise them to patients but ethical to advertise them to physicians.

Since prescription drugs include the great majority of all remedies, since they are monitored for years before they can be sold directly to the public, and since serious adverse reactions are more likely to occur following their use, they are far more important from medical, public health, and regulatory standpoints than those sold over the counter. For these reasons, this book will be confined to a consideration of prescription drugs.

When medicines are pure, when they are effective, when

enough is known about them, and when they are wisely selected and properly taken, they mean better health for everyone. This is reflected in the relative freedom from discomfort and disease of the average man and woman today; it is also reflected in the statistics of the past century, which show diminishing death rates and increasing length of life for the people of every country where modern drugs, along with the knowledge of how to use them, are available. To be sure, lowered death rates are caused in part by improved sanitation and other public health measures, in part by improved nutrition, and in part by other factors. Yet the steepened slope of the downward curve of the death rate for many infections since the advent of chemotherapy, and the almost complete absence of certain infectious diseases from our hospitals in recent years, show that the newer remedies have had their own dramatic effects.

On the other hand, drugs may produce discomfort, disability, or even death. These adverse reactions, although sometimes unavoidable, can often be prevented when doctors are knowledgeable and alert.

The good health that stems from good drugs properly used, and the ill health that can follow from misuse, give medicines a social as well as an individual significance. Each new drug successfully developed fosters hope and feeds demand for more successes. Society is thus concerned, because scientific knowledge and technical competence of the highest order are required to originate, produce, use, and judge the effects of drugs; society must provide the trained professionals to do these things.

Medicines have economic significance because of the complicated and expensive apparatus and machinery required for innovating, manufacturing, processing, and testing them. Making drugs is big business; those manufactured in this country in 1965 were valued at over three and one-half billion dollars.[1] Their broad social and economic impact forces the government to become involved. Thus drugs permeate the body social and the body political, just as they permeate the body physical. This book will be concerned with these interrelationships.

Technological change requires social change; this in turn

demands more technological change. These recurring cycles are the wheels that carry mankind forward. They revolve upon the axle of knowledge, which in recent centuries has been scientific knowledge, and are powered by man's desire for a better life. Nowhere is this pattern more evident than in the process of bringing drugs to the point where they are given to people to prevent or cure disease.

The frontispiece illustrates how a drug was prepared in the sixteenth century—in this case guaiac, which was at that time in vogue as the treatment for syphilis. In one room, a servant is chipping a huge log, another is weighing the chips, and a third is making an infusion from them. In the other room, the infusion is being given directly to the patient. Incidentally, along with this simplicity in method went a credulousness in judgment. All the work of the servants, all the urgings of the doctor, and all the gagging of the bitter potion on the part of the poor patient went for naught. Guaiac, despite the meaning of its name—"holy wood"—was utterly worthless as a treatment for syphilis.

In contrast, many and diverse groups involved in the discovery, production, regulation, and use of drugs today can be seen in Figure 1. Research and discovery, which originate them, take place mostly in the laboratories of pharmaceutical companies, universities, and government. The technological development of chemical compounds and substances derived from plant and animal sources into the best products for human consumption, and the fashioning of the finished products, occur today almost entirely in industrial plants. The primary substances and the finished products are tested in laboratories and in animals by industrial and university scientists. The final products are tested in humans by physicians or other practitioners. Then they must pass the fine screen of government review. For most drugs this means the Food and Drug Administration of the federal government; in the case of serums and vaccines the responsibility rests with the National Institutes of Health. Some state governments impose additional controls. After this the drugs are promoted, distributed, and sold by the pharmaceutical companies and by wholesalers and pharmacists, although some are purchased by governments and hospitals for direct distribution and use.

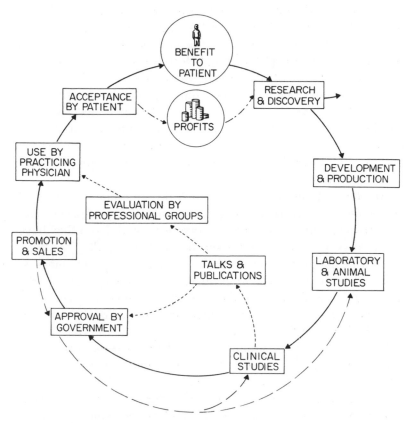

Figure 1. Pathway of a drug from discovery to eventual use.

Meanwhile physician-investigators who have studied the new drugs are telling their colleagues about them, person to person, in speeches to groups, in medical journals, and in books. Certain professional organizations, such as the Council on Drugs of the American Medical Association and the United States Pharmacopeial Convention, evaluate their effectiveness, safety, and usefulness and publish these evaluations. The combined effects of the advertising and the observations and opinions of professional colleagues determine the extent and nature of the use of the drug by the practicing physician.

The Food and Drug Administration has a further check. It

monitors the labeling and advertising of each drug and may require that they be changed, just as it may require further testing of a drug in the laboratory or in patients. Finally, of course, the patient must accept the drug before it can be used. He must purchase the prescribed medicine and take each dose, or he must permit someone to give it to him, by injection or otherwise. When all of these steps are taken, it is expected that the drug will benefit the patient and bring profits to the producer. Both of these motives supply the impetus for further research, for the discovery of other drugs—in other words, they supply the force that starts the cycle over again.

In the past the public has paid little attention to the social and economic effects of drugs, and only the professions and industries directly involved have been interested. Even they have not always looked beyond their noses. Periodically, however, enough people become aroused about the safety, purity, efficacy, availability, or price of drugs to make drastic changes in the laws regulating them. Three times in this country, in 1906, 1938, and 1962, the storm clouds of popular opinion have thundered over the heads of the regulated and have resulted in drastic new federal laws on drugs. Following each law has come a period of adjustment, but the onward rush of technology has made each rebalancing only a precarious prelude to another imbalance.

We are at present in a time of turbulence, attempting to adapt to the 1962 Drug Amendments Act and at the same time questioning whether this law will solve our problem of getting the right drug in its right form to the right person at the right time at the right price. Many people are unsure. As Seymour E. Harris says:

"Drugs have become a hot issue in medicine. The large outlays, the high prices, the Kefauver hearings in the Senate with their emphasis on monopoly practice, excessive profits and selling costs, some evidence of dishonest and misleading advertising and the resultant proposals for new legislation; the increasing contribution of drugs to the saving of lives and shortening of hospital stays, the rising significance of prescription medicine against purchases over the counter—all of these have increased interest in the drug industry."[2]

Certainly, to assume that all the problems are solved because we now have a law on the books would be carelessly complacent and incredibly naive. Even though administered by the wisest of men, the Drug Amendments Act of 1962 can touch only a few of the technological, social, and economic problems affected by drugs. But some problems the law does not directly affect: the need for more research, for better teaching in medical schools, for self-regulation by the health professions, for more knowledge on the part of doctors, and for more participation in decision-making by the patient and the public.

When technological change produces social change, it splits opinion. Nowhere has this happened more than in the drug field. Some believe that the executives of the drug industry have contributed more to human happiness in the twentieth century than any group of similar size. Others would say of them (as Shakespeare said of Coriolanus) that they:

> *. . . did*
> *Run reeking o'er the lives of men, as if*
> *'Twere a perpetual spoil.*

Some think of government officials who regulate drugs as the highest type of public servant; others consider them nit-pickers, afraid to make a decision, afraid even of their own shadows. Some, along with Robert Louis Stevenson, think of practicing doctors as the flower of our civilization; others think of them as dupes, easily led by a few seductive words to give drugs carelessly, often to no benefit and sometimes to the harm of their patients.

A much less discussed area, but one of equal importance, is the adequacy of the physician's knowledge about drugs and how he applies it. Criticism has been leveled at medical schools for not teaching enough about drug therapy, at doctors for not keeping up with the latest knowledge, at government agencies for not co-ordinating information and placing it at the doctors' fingertips, and at drug companies for obscuring the known facts in a fog of advertising. Others excuse deficiencies by citing the crowded curriculums of the medical schools, which prohibit spending too much time on any one subject, and the shortage of doctors, who thus are forced to see an extra dozen or so patients instead of reading or attending a medical meeting. The defenders of the drug industry claim that it does yeoman service in bridging the information gap with its advertising and its educational programs. And so goes the debate. It seems that we can agree on only one thing: that there is no agreement.

Differences of opinion such as these can be tackled in two ways. The adversary method permits each side in the controversy to marshal the facts and opinions that it thinks will win its point, and to arm itself with the strongest of words, often the most barbed epithets that can be found. Those facts that do not forward the argument are pushed out of sight or buried in a fog of debate. This is the method that many believe was used by the several congressional subcommittees that have in the last few years inquired into the pricing and regulation of drugs and the dissemination of information about them. It has also been used by spokesmen for industry, both as witnesses in these hearings and in speeches and articles directed toward the medical profession and the public. Authors of several recent books on the regulation of drugs have also employed the adversary method.

In a Few Hands[3] is the late Senator Estes Kefauver's own story of the hearings on monopoly held by a Senate subcommittee of which he was chairman, and discusses particularly the drug, automobile, steel, and bakery industries. Richard Harris in *The Real Voice*[4] concentrates on the events leading up to the passage of the Drug Amendments Act of 1962, casting Senator Kefauver in the role of the man on the white horse. *By Prescription Only*, by Morton Mintz,[5] uses material from the hearings of several congressional committees to accuse not only the pharmaceutical industry but also organized medicine and at times the federal Food and Drug Administration of neglecting the consumers' interests. This method has its advantages. Without doubt, congressional hearings and the speeches, articles and books that speak for a special group or a particular philosophy, have uncovered important facts, set forth worth-while opinions, and goaded people into action.

Yet I believe the time has come for persons in the health

professions to utilize the other, the scientific, method in judging how well drugs are developed, tested, and used. In this method the observer scrutinizes and sifts the many facts and diverse opinions, weighs and balances them, and reaches a judgment that is as free of emotion and self-interest as possible. Granted that these can never be completely eliminated, and granted that no one can set himself to be the sole judge of issues so important to life and health and happiness, to scientific progress, and to individual liberty; yet only by attempting to reach balanced judgments can we hope to see clearly what we have done, what we are doing, and what we need to do. Believing, with Jacques Barzun,[6] that dealing solely with the contemporary, by shortening judgment and distorting perspective, prepares one poorly to think an important matter through, I have tried to dig to the historical roots of the institutions and movements involved. I am sure that my conclusions will not be universally agreed with, but I hope that some of them will become a common ground on which all parties may meet to plan the further advance of their mutual interests.

In gathering the facts and in offering suggestions, I have been concerned primarily with improvements that will advance the health of the American people. Economic considerations force themselves into any study of drug innovation, production, regulation, or use, but they must be kept in second place. For in the long run, as Alan Gregg said, ". . . the profits of medical research could be audited only by an expert accountant for the human race, an expert accountant in suffering and in health, now and in the long future."[7]

1

The Discovery
of Drugs

To understand the present and plan the future we need to know how today's abundance of drugs evolved. In this chapter I shall discuss what is generally called the discovery of drugs. Sometimes drugs are actually stumbled upon—literally dis-covered. More often, especially in recent years, they are invented; new chemical or biological entities are created and then tested for preventive or therapeutic effects. But the word "discovery" is so commonly used to describe both discovery and invention that I shall use it to mean finding or devising a new therapeutic or prophylactic substance.

New drugs have sometimes been discovered by individuals—physicians or laymen—working alone, but more often in the laboratories of universities, research institutes, pharmaceutical companies, or government. The relative importance of these individuals and groups has changed from time to time as the result of several clearly definable trends: the increased number of effective drugs that have become available, especially in recent years; the shift in the source of drugs, from nature-made to man-made; new methods used to discover drugs; the increased effectiveness of today's remedies over yesterday's; and changed methods of administering drugs.

Less than two dozen effective drugs were known before the year 1700. Among these were the cathartics, senna, aloe, figs, and castor oil. The purgative effects of the last were known to Herodotus. Intestinal worms, a common problem in tropical countries and in unsanitary environments, were combated by the roots of aspidium (male fern), by the bark from the pomegranate tree, by an oil expressed from the flowers of santonin (Levant wormseed), or by an oil from the fruit and leaves of chenopodium (American wormseed). The first three originated in the Orient and the Near East; the last was used by the American Indians. Mercury was used as a purgative, as a diuretic, and later also as a specific remedy for syphilis.

Alcohol, opium, and the leaves of the hyoscyamus plant were employed for centuries to induce sleep and relieve pain. The last contains scopolamine, which until recently was used, along with morphine, to diminish the pains of childbirth. This combination produced the so-called twilight sleep, in which pain and consciousness were blunted and the patient had no memory of events afterward.

The Arabs in the sixteenth century began to use colchicum, derived from the stem of the meadow saffron, for rheumatic pains; eventually it was found to be a specific remedy for acute attacks of gout. Other specific remedies in use before 1700 were: for malaria, cinchona bark, the source of quinine; for amoebic dysentery, ipecac, the root of a Brazilian plant, ipecacuanha; and for leprosy, chaulmoogra oil, obtained from the seeds of certain East Indian trees.

A number of drugs were used as tonics. Among them were iron, which we now know will speed recovery in anemia caused by loss of blood, and nux vomica, the source of strychnine, which had such a bitter taste that it stimulated the appetite.

Other drugs were used for a while and forgotten. Arab physicians in the twelfth century gave burned sponge to shrink goiters; and though it was effective, presumably because of its iodine content, the reason for its use was not understood and the practice was never widespread. That iodine would cure goiter had to be rediscovered in the nineteenth century. Likewise, ergot was used by midwives to contract the uterus at least as early as the sixteenth century, but it was not officially accepted by physicians until 1808.

The few effective drugs that were known were used alongside many other substances that were either valueless or downright poisonous, and so many drugs were mixed in a single prescription that we have to strain our credulity to believe that physicians usually knew when they were using an effective remedy and when they were not. The ancient Egyptians, while they used opium for pain, castor oil and senna as cathartics, and pomegranate to rid the intestines of worms, also prescribed a mixture of writing ink and cerebrospinal fluid for baldness and compounded their drugs with blood, viscera, and excreta of animals. Similar nauseous mixtures were trustingly imbibed by patients not only in ancient times but through the Middle Ages. Even at the end of the seventeenth century, Robert Boyle, who helped lay the scientific basis of modern chemistry, treated his patients with powdered cow dung for infection of the eyes. And although some specific remedies—drugs with special effects in the prevention or cure of a particular disease—were available, their value was not always appreciated. During the sixteenth century guaiac came into vogue for the treatment of syphilis, temporarily displacing mercury, which had definite curative effects, although guaiac will neither cure syphilis nor abate its symptoms in the slightest degree.

The ferment of the Renaissance and the pursuit of science began to pay off for therapeutics in the eighteenth century. Four events were of special importance. Variolation, the practice of inoculating nonimmune persons from the pustules of smallpox to produce a slight local infection that would protect against developing the generalized disease, was introduced into England in 1721. James Lind's *A Treatise of the Scurvy* appeared in 1753, describing his carefully controlled experiments that demonstrated beyond doubt that adding citrus fruits to sailors' diets cured scurvy. This was the first insight into the mystery of vitamins. In 1785 William Withering published his book *An Account of the Foxglove and Some of Its Medical Uses*, which described the actions of digitalis on patients so accurately that clinical observation in the intervening centuries has added practically nothing more. And finally, this epoch-making century closed with Edward Jenner's demonstration that vaccination, inoculation with cowpox, would prevent smallpox.

The nineteenth century was marked by several milestones. It started with the isolation of alkaloids, organic chemical substances, alkaline in reaction, found in plants. The first was morphine, obtained from crude opium. Others were atropine (from belladonna), caffeine (from coffee and tea), nicotine (from tobacco), quinine (from cinchona bark), and strychnine (from nux vomica). The extraction of these active principles not only made the drug available in pure form and in measurable quantities; more important, the therapeutic properties of the drug could be studied accurately and any adverse effects could be clearly attributed to it. Finally, as we shall see later, the production of substances that were potent in minute amounts demanded rigid control of quality, quantity, and purity. Today the practice of isolating the active principle of a drug is so routine that we tend to forget what an important step it was.

The next significant advance was a happy combination of chemical invention and clinical observation. Chemists had made a number of substances that later turned out to have anesthetic properties, but not until 1846 was one of them, ether, first shown conclusively to have this effect. At about the same time nitrous oxide and chloroform were shown to be anesthetics, too, and a door was opened through which dozens of anesthetics have been introduced since.

Yet in spite of these advances, progress was all too slow. In the middle of the eighteenth century, medicine was still sneeringly referred to as the withered arm of science, and in 1860 Oliver Wendell Holmes wrote of his firm belief that with the exception of opium, the anesthetics, and a few specifics, "if the whole *materia medica*, as now used, could be sunk to the bottom of the sea, it would be all the better for mankind—and all the worse for the fishes."[1]

The date has ironic significance because in that same year coal tar was used to synthesize salicylic acid, the first drug that was a by-product of research on dyes. The synthesis of aspirin, antipyrine, phenacetin, and dozens of other drugs followed. Thus, by the end of the nineteenth century the extraction of the active principles of drugs and the synthesis of new chemical substances were firmly established as the twin pillars upon which modern pharmaceutical chemistry is based.

The science of bacteriology began with the researches of Koch and Pasteur around 1860. Its first fruits appeared in 1881, when Pasteur made a vaccine against anthrax by weakening the micro-organisms so that when they were injected they would no longer cause disease but would still produce immunity. He used this method even more dramatically when he made a rabies vaccine and gave it with success to a severely bitten child in

1885. Before the end of the century effective vaccines had been developed for typhoid fever, cholera, and plague.

Research had also shown that some bacteria manufactured toxins, substances that injured the tissues of the host (animal or human). The host, in turn, generated substances called antitoxins, which neutralized the toxins. Antitoxins were produced by injecting the toxins of bacteria into animals and under sterile conditions collecting the serum, which could then be given to a patient who had the disease. Antitoxin against diphtheria was first made in 1889, followed in a few years by tetanus antitoxin. Unfortunately, most bacterial infections are not caused by toxins, and the perfection of antiserums to neutralize whole bacteria had to wait until the next century.

By the end of the nineteenth century these discoveries were having their effect. The Eighth Revision of *The United States Pharmacopeia* (*USP*) published in 1905, contained (in addition to⸱ a number of cathartics) digitalis, quinine, ipecac, caffeine, mercury, and iron; the anesthetics: ether, chloroform, and cocaine; and several pain-relieving drugs and sedatives: morphine, codeine, salicylates, acetanilid, phenacetin, chloral, and the bromides. The remaining drugs, about two hundred of them, were either worthless or had only a minor therapeutic effect. The research of three centuries on the basic sciences that undergird medicine was paying off in increased understanding of disease, in better methods of diagnosing disease, and in furthering the public health, but therapeutics had been only lightly touched as yet.[2]

The seeds had been sown, and the real harvest came in the twentieth century. Because it was so abundant, I have divided the important drugs introduced in this century into four groups according to their derivation (Table 1). Extraction of animal tissue produced a few of the twentieth century drugs; a great many more were synthesized. Vaccines were perfected to prevent, and serums to treat, a number of infectious diseases. These are called biologicals because they are produced by biological rather than chemical methods. Finally, the field of antibiotics was opened.

The drugs listed are only those that represent the opening

of a door to a new class of compounds. Soon after a new drug is perfected, dozens of compounds with nearly identical chemical structure are often synthesized. These are called analogues (or, somewhat sarcastically, "me-too" drugs). They tend to displace the initial drug in the group, because they are more effective therapeutically, cause fewer adverse effects, can be produced more cheaply, or are marketed with a more aggressive advertising campaign. For instance, the extraction of adrenal cortex in 1929, the synthesis in 1937 of desoxycorticosterone, which had some of the actions of the adrenal cortex, and the extraction in 1949 of cortisone, the active principle of the adrenal cortex, were followed by the synthesis of several analogues that displaced the originals. Likewise, soon after the male and female hormones, androsterone and estrogenic hormones, were isolated, many similar substances were produced by chemical synthesis. In the same way, barbital was followed by other barbiturates; epinephrine by other drugs that act on the sympathetic nervous system, such as ephedrine and amphetamine.

The idea that if one looked hard enough, one could find for any bacterium or protozoan a chemical substance that, when attached to the micro-organism, would knock it out of commission, was at first only a glimmer in the mind of Paul Ehrlich. But by following this idea, Ehrlich made atoxyl, the first effective drug against trypanosomiasis, or African sleeping sickness. More important were arsphenamine and neoarsphenamine produced in 1909 and 1912 respectively; these became the mainstay of the therapy of syphilis until penicillin was discovered.

The discovery of the effectiveness of plasmoquin started an intensive hunt for other synthetics of related chemical structure. How these were found and tested under the pressure of World War II forms one of the most fascinating chapters in the history of that war.[3]

In 1932 Gerhard Domagk made a discovery in the laboratories of the I. G. Farbenindustrie of Germany that won him a Nobel Prize. He found that Prontosil rubrum, a red dye with a complicated chemical formula, protected animals from streptococcal infections. After three more years of animal and clinical trials

TABLE 1. **Important Drugs Introduced Into Medical Practice After 1900**

Drugs Obtained by Extraction	Drugs Obtained by Synthesis	Biologicals	Antibiotics
	1903 Barbital (first of the barbiturates)		
	1904 Epinephrine (first hormone to be synthesized)		
	1905 Atoxyl (for trypanosomiasis)	1905 Antimeningococcic serum	
	1909 Arsphenamine (for syphilis)		
1918 Heparin (anti-coagulant)			
1921 Insulin (for diabetes)			
	1923 Tetanus toxoid		
	1926 Plasmoquin (for malaria)		
1929 Adrenal cortex			
1929 Estrogenic hormone		1930 Typhus vaccine	
1931 Androsterone			
1931 *Rauwolfia serpentina* (first drug effective against high blood pressure; source of reserpine)	1932 Prontosil patented (first sulfa drug)		

Drugs Obtained by Extraction	Drugs Obtained by Synthesis	Biologicals	Antibiotics
	1937 Desoxycorticosterone (for Addison's disease)		
	1938 Diphenylhydantoin (for epilepsy)		
	1939 Bishydroxycoumarin (first oral anticoagulant)		
	1942 Antergan (first antihistaminic)		1942 Penicillin first prepared
	1942 Nitrogen mustard (first drug effective against malignant tumors)		
			1944 Streptomycin
			1948 Chlortetracycline
1949 Cortisone (for rheumatoid arthritis)			
	1952 Chlorpromazine (first of tranquilizers)		
		1954 Poliomyelitis vaccine	1954 Nystatin (first antifungal antibiotic)
	1955 Sulfonylureas (oral antidiabetic agents)		
			1960 Methicillin
	1963 Idoxuridine (first antiviral drug)		

he announced the discovery. The next year French investigators reported that the complex dye was not essential, that the effective component was sulfanilamide. Since this relatively simple substance was not patented, doctors all over the world were free to use it. More important still, chemists could modify it easily. Numerous derivatives were synthesized until compounds were found that were effective in a larger group of diseases and caused fewer adverse effects than sulfanilamide, and new ones are still being synthesized today. The sulfa drugs also stimulated the search for other synthetics for use in bacterial infections. This produced isoniazid, which was as great a contribution to tuberculosis control as the sulfonamides were to streptococcal infections, and several drugs of lesser importance for various bacterial infections. It also stimulated a hunt for antiviral drugs—a hunt so prolonged that many thought it hopeless until in 1963 idoxuridine was found to accelerate the cure of infections of the eye caused by the *herpes simplex* virus (the fever blister virus). Two other and totally different antiviral drugs followed: methisazone, which has some preventive effect against smallpox, and amantadine, against some types of influenza. While these three drugs are not highly effective themselves, they appear to me to herald the day when antiviral drugs will be as effective and as numerous as the many antibacterial drugs now in use.

After nitrogen mustard, which had been used as a gas during World War I, was found to be effective against some forms of cancer, the push was on to find others, of which methotrexate appears to be the first drug that has actually cured any form of cancer. The story of the anti-epileptic, antihistaminic, and anticoagulant drugs and the tranquilizers is similar: the first was found; then dozens of others followed.

Among the biologicals, a serum against the meningococcus, the cause of the most common type of meningitis, was the first serum that was effective against whole bacteria, but its importance was overshadowed by the serum against the pneumococcus, the most frequent cause of pneumonia. This was perfected in the 1920's and 1930's and used extensively in several state-wide programs.

Typhus vaccine was the first one effective against the rickettsial organisms, which are tiny bacteria that resemble viruses in that they grow only within cells. Tetanus toxoid was the first effective vaccine against a toxin-producing disease, tetanus. Poliomyelitis vaccine was the first vaccine to be made from viruses grown in tissues in the incubator, rather than in intact animals or eggs. It opened the way for vaccines against measles and rubella (German measles) and, I hope, before long, the common cold.

The antibiotics included in Table 1 are those that marked the greatest steps forward: penicillin, the first safe and effective antibiotic; streptomycin, the first one effective against tuberculosis; chlortetracycline, the first broad-spectrum antibiotic; nystatin, the first antibiotic effective against fungi; and methicillin, the first semisynthetic analogue of penicillin to cure infections caused by staphylococci resistant to penicillin itself. Here also, when a door was opened by one drug, other drugs followed. Several antibiotics and several chemicals are now used to treat tuberculosis; a half-dozen broad-spectrum antibiotics are on the market; two more antifungal antibiotics followed nystatin, and there are now several semisynthetic penicillins and probably many more to come.

A second trend in the past hundred years is change in the sources of drugs. Among the 286 therapeutic or preventive drugs listed in the 1965 Seventeenth Revision of the *USP* (excluding duplicate salts of identical substances), 179 (or 63 per cent) were synthetic organic chemicals and 19 (or 7 per cent) were of vegetable origin. This can be contrasted with the 80 per cent of drugs of vegetable origin in the Fourth Revision of the *USP*, published about one hundred years ago. Among these were many that were worthless as drugs, such as wormwood, camomile, pipsissewa, isinglass, oak bark, and tobacco. This *USP* contained no synthetics, and even a half century later, in the 1916 edition, only 11 per cent of all the drugs were synthetics.

By 1868, the percentage of drugs from animal sources had

fallen to its lowest point. The *USP* had been purged of filth. It no longer contained ants, earthworms, grasshoppers, the excrements of pigeons, the tails of lizards, or the eyes of crayfish, which were among the many items listed in the *Pharmacopoeia Londinensis* of 1618.[4] In the 1916 edition, drugs from animal sources were coming back, but they were based on rational therapeutics. The most important were thyroid gland, cod liver oil, which remained for many years the best source of vitamins A and D, and pepsin from the stomach secretions. By 1965, extracts from the parathyroid and pituitary glands had been added; heparin, from the liver, to delay the clotting of blood; and insulin and glucagon for the regulation of the concentration of glucose in the blood.

Moreover, the drugs from animal sources in the 1916 *USP* were either of low potency or altogether worthless; those in the 1965 edition are highly active extracts obtained by sophisticated methods, and their potency is carefully evaluated by chemical assays or by injecting them into animals and determining the quantity that will kill the animals or the effect of different quantities on individual organs and tissues.

Biologicals were just beginning to be produced at the start of the century; since then, the number, variety, and effectiveness of serums and vaccines have steadily increased. The techniques that had been developed in perfecting the serums of lower animals began to be used to preserve fractions of human blood and other tissues. These are used mostly to combat infections (for instance, immune globulin for measles and infectious hepatitis) and to promote the coagulation of blood. And of course the antibiotics represent a whole new group of drugs unknown before penicillin. They are mostly prepared by fermentation methods, although a few are synthesized.

The change in the sources of drugs fostered a third trend in the past century: a shift in the method of innovating. When drugs came mostly from natural sources, the physician usually discovered their value in the treatment of disease, and either he or a pharmacist experimented with the best methods of insuring uniform dosage. This method of finding new drugs has become less and less productive, although there are a few recent examples: the discovery by Minot and Murphy of Boston in 1926 that liver contained a substance that was missing in patients with pernicious anemia and if given periodically would keep them in perfect health; the demonstration in the early 1950's by an Indian physician named Vakil that the root of *Rauwolfia serpentina*, a shrub found in the Orient from India to Sumatra, would lower high blood pressure. Later, reserpine was extracted from this plant.

When observations on the effects of natural substances were combined with the increasing skills of the chemists, there followed a more sophisticated method of originating a drug: extracting from the natural product the portion having the pharmacological effect. This meant more exact control of the purity and the dose of drugs. Examples are the use of morphine instead of crude opium, quinine instead of cinchona, or reserpine instead of *Rauwolfia serpentina*. The next step in the history of drug discovery was to determine the chemical formula of an extract and, if possible, synthesize it. Epinephrine was originally extracted from the suprarenal gland, and the antibiotic, chloramphenicol, was first made by fermentation; today they are synthesized, because this can be done more cheaply. Thus, while premodern man looked around him for drugs, modern man fashions his own.

Once the chemical composition is known, it can often be changed in the laboratory. This has been called molecular manipulation, but the term has a pejorative connotation that is not deserved. "Molecular improvement" is preferable. Changes in the molecule often lead to a better drug. Prontosil and sulfanilamide were not effective in pneumococcal infections; sulfapyridine was. Sulfadiazine acted against an even wider range of bacterial infections and at the same time caused fewer side reactions than sulfapyridine.

An analogue may produce fewer or less severe adverse reactions than the original drug. Thus, tetracycline caused fewer gastrointestinal symptoms than the original drug in the series, chlortetracycline. Sometimes a change in the molecule improves or delays absorption. Penicillin V, which is made from the original penicillin G by changing only one end of a long molecule, is absorbed better than the original, especially after meals. On the other hand, sulfaguanidine and succinylsulfathiazole were devised as modifications of sulfanilamide because they were absorbed little, if at all, and thus would remain in the gastrointestinal tract to suppress the growth of bacteria. They have been used extensively by surgeons before operations in which the intestines are to be opened.

Sometimes the newer analogues are more potent than the original. For instance, 20 mg. of hydrocortisone, 5 mg. of prednisone, 4 mg. of triamcinolone, and 0.75 mg. of dexamethasone have the same therapeutic action as 25 mg. of the original cortisone. Here we encounter the problem of whether such an increase in potency has any significance. Greater potency may mean fewer side reactions, but frequently the more potent analogue causes as many adverse reactions as the original and sometimes even more. In such cases the increased potency is significant only if the price of the more active drug is low enough so that the patient pays less for the same therapeutic result. Unfortunately, as we shall see later, this is not usually the case.

This brings us to a second class of analogues: those that represent no real improvement over similar drugs that are already well established in use. Examples include many of the sulfa drugs, the barbiturates, the tranquilizers, and the antihistaminics.

Finally, we come to the most important reason for modifying the chemical structure of a drug: sometimes a drug is produced that has actions entirely different from the original drug. The observation, made in 1942, that sulfanilamide lowered the blood sugar was ignored at the time, but when one of its analogues, carbutamide, originally developed for use in infections, was found to have a pronounced effect on the blood sugar, an active search for similar compounds began. The result was a safer drug, tolbutamide, which has enabled thousands of people with diabetes to control this disease without resorting to insulin.

An even more striking example was the finding that a minor

chemical modification of morphine would produce a major pharmacological result. This modification, nalorphine, antagonizes many of the physiological effects of morphine, codeine, and related drugs, such as depression of respiration, low blood pressure, and coma. Thus it can save the life of someone who has had an overdose of one of these drugs. It is also used to diagnose and treat narcotics addicts.

Today changing the molecules of drugs of known effectiveness is the most common method of looking for new drugs. In addition there are two others. Screening a large number of compounds that have been synthesized for other purposes is employed especially in the search for antibiotics and anticancer drugs. The number of compounds that have been screened is fantastic: 10,000 sulfonamides, 25,000 antimalarials, 30,000 antituberculous agents, and 125,000 compounds developed in the search for a cancer cure.[5] Considering all the time and money that the screening takes (estimated at $2,000 for each compound screened), it has not been a particularly productive method. Yet it sometimes yields unexpected dividends, as in the case of an important antihypertensive drug, guanethidine, which was discovered by screening new compounds thought to be of value in trypanosomal infections.[6]

Finally, there is the theoretical method of devising new drugs. Basic research in physiology tells us how the body works; from this we can sometimes deduce how its actions can be modified. One example was the work on penicillin by Karl Beyer and associates of Merck Sharp & Dohme. Because this antibiotic is excreted so rapidly through the kidneys, large doses have to be given. Some wag likened this to trying to fill a bathtub without putting in the stopper. It was known that penicillin was excreted through the tubules of the kidneys. Therefore, reasoned these investigators, if another substance that was excreted through these tubules were given at the same time, the excretion of penicillin ought to be delayed. The first drug they used, para-aminohippuric acid, did slow the excretion of penicillin, but was itself excreted so fast that large doses were needed.[7] Probing further, they synthesized probenecid, which would do the trick in much smaller doses. Later, probenecid was shown to increase the excretion of uric acid by the kidneys and thus also became an important drug in the treatment of gout.

Serums and vaccines are examples of drugs made on the basis of theoretical principles. The discoveries of Pasteur, Koch, and their pupils led to the hope that a vaccine or serum could be developed to prevent or cure every infectious disease. Although serums against diphtheria, tetanus, and pneumococcal pneumonia were highly effective and several other less so, serum therapy on the whole did not fulfill its original promise. Vaccines against smallpox, diphtheria, tetanus, and typhoid fever were highly effective; others such as BCG vaccine for tuberculosis had restricted usefulness; and other suspensions of bacteria, such as those that were purported to abort the common cold, just didn't work at all. Recently, following the growth of viruses in tissue culture, there has been a resurgence of interest in vaccines against viral infections, with success in vaccines against poliomyelitis and measles and more to come.

While microbiology gives promise of developing drugs on a theoretical basis, in the chemical field the theoretical method has yielded very few drugs, although many believe that it will eventually be the most productive method. At present the cost of beginning with a theoretical idea and following it through all its ramifications in the hope of originating a drug is so high as to be prohibitive except in an area of great need such as cancer, and here the large sums expended have not paid off as yet.

The methods that are now used to find new drugs require expertly trained workers, sophisticated instruments, and complex machinery. As a result the innovator of a new drug today is seldom the practicing physician, but rather a group of investigators in the laboratory of a university, a drug firm, or a government. This change will be discussed in more detail in Chapter 2.

A fourth trend is the increasing effectiveness of today's drugs. Although some of the drugs in use for centuries are still in the doctor's armamentarium, most have been replaced by better ones. The improvement has sometimes consisted of using the active principle, as digitalis glycosides instead of digitalis, emetine instead of ipecac, quinine instead of cinchona bark, morphine instead of opium. More often it has meant a shift to a better analogue made synthetically, as aspirin (acetylsalicylic acid) instead of the salicylic acid obtained from willow bark, or prednisone instead of the cortisone extracted from the adrenal gland.

In other cases, a totally unrelated drug has been found superior to the original in therapeutic action and has displaced it, as chloroquin instead of quinine in malaria, or the shifts in the treatment of pneumococcic infections and syphilis. In the treatment of syphilis, arsphenamine and other arsenicals have replaced mercury, but penicillin made them all obsolete almost overnight. In pneumococcic pneumonia, before specific treatment was available one third of the patients died. Serums that acted against the pneumococci reduced the fatality rate to 16.7 per cent; sulfa drugs displaced serums because they lowered the rate to 12.3 per cent, but they were displaced in turn by penicillin and the tetracyclines, which dropped the death rate to 5.1 per cent.[8]

More important still, new drugs have opened therapeutic doors where mankind had faced a blank wall. Some of the most dramatic of these breakthroughs were the discovery of insulin for diabetes mellitus, liver for pernicious anemia, penicillin for bacterial endocarditis, streptomycin and isoniazid for tuberculosis, and a number of drugs that arrest the growth of cancer cells.

Thus the modern doctor has available dozens of potent drugs that have displaced the crude, the inferior, and the worthless drugs his predecessors used a hundred, fifty, or even ten years ago. This is the opposite of Gresham's law; the good drugs drive out the bad. One proof of the trend toward better and better drugs is the fact that among the 286 individual drugs in the Seventeenth Revision of the *USP* published in 1965, two thirds have been introduced since 1900, and a similar number of worthless or outmoded drugs have been discarded.

A fifth trend is the administration of drugs by new routes. In the remote past people thought drugs would work if they were applied locally; now we know that absorption through the skin is limited, so that drugs are applied locally mainly for diseases of the skin or other accessible areas, or for caustic effects on tumors. Taking drugs by mouth has, of course, always been the most convenient route and still is. But in the past fifty years, subcutaneous and especially intravenous methods have displaced the oral route when exact doses or large amounts are needed or when vomiting or coma precludes taking the drug by mouth. Before these routes were used extensively, doctors tried with indifferent success to give drugs by rectum, and while this method is still used, especially for patients outside the hospital, it has been largely superseded by subcutaneous and intravenous injection. Finally, the method of inhalation has been gradually refined and is being explored for drugs other than the anesthetics.

In summary, effective new drugs have been introduced at an ever-accelerating rate; today in contrast to the past they come from different sources, such as synthetic chemicals, serums, vaccines, and antibiotics; innovation of drugs occurs mostly by changing the configurations of molecules; this year's drugs on the whole are better than last year's, and those in turn better than the drugs of a decade ago, and still better than those of a century ago; finally, an increasing percentage of drugs is given subcutaneously, intravenously, and by inhalation.

Formerly the industry made what the physician prescribed; now the physician prescribes what the industry makes.
—Report by the Committee
on Public Health,
New York Academy of Medicine

2

Institutionalization of the Research and Development of Drugs

Man has discovered some drugs by stumbling upon them, but at the rate he was going up to 1800 it would have taken him several millennia to stock the shelves of today's drugstore, assuming he would ever have reached that point. In drug-making, as in transportation, power, communications, and the exploration of space, man has accelerated the conquest of nature by developing the process of innovation. He has, as Alfred North Whitehead says, invented the method of invention. In the process research on drugs and their development to a marketable state have become institutionalized. The shift from natural substances to products of the chemical and bacteriological laboratories, the screening of hundreds of compounds to find one that is effective, and the accelerating pace of discovery have demanded teams of highly trained workers. These could be found only in institutions. Such an institution might have other interests, as in the case of a university, a research institute, or a government laboratory; or it might be established specifically to produce drugs—a pharmaceutical company.

Basic research and technological development are, of course, not the same thing. Science wants to acquire knowledge; technology, to use it. But the exact point at which science leaves off and technology begins is always a good subject for an hour's argument. Especially in producing new drugs, research and development are so closely allied that they are best considered together. The special incentives and pressures of each will be evident as individual examples are taken up.

Research laboratories in universities made a slow and faltering start in Italy in the fourteenth century, but the modern research laboratory really began in Germany in the late eighteenth century and was full-blown by the nineteenth. In that country a few physicians, seeing that the medicine of the day had too little to offer to the patient, turned their backs on practice and gave their lives to research. At first the subjects that absorbed them were anatomy, physiology, pathology, and chemistry; but the study of the normal and diseased body eventually led to the study of how its actions might be modified by drugs; in other words, pharmacology. During the latter half of the nineteenth century the German universities trained men who established departments of pharmacology all over the world. There were no separate departments of pharmacology in English medical schools in 1900; by 1960 there were nineteen.[1] In 1968 there were eighty-one independent departments of pharmacology in the eighty-six medical schools in the United States.[2]

The other of the twin pillars of drug research—microbiology —was recognized by the creation of independent laboratories soon after Pasteur and Koch established it as a science. A bacteriological laboratory was set up for Koch in the Imperial Health Office in 1880 and a professorship created for him at the University of Berlin in 1885. France likewise honored its hero by establishing the Pasteur Institute in 1888. These were followed by institutes in other countries. Meanwhile departments of bacteriology or microbiology were established in most medical schools and elsewhere in universities, and they took over the job of training the newcomers to the profession as well as a great part of the research.

Most of the contributions to our knowledge of the physiological properties of drugs, such as their action on the heart, the lungs, the kidneys, and the central nervous system, their action on individual cells, and their passage through cell membranes, have come from university laboratories. But some of the research in universities has also been directed toward producing new drugs. Among the Nobel Prize winners from universities have been George R. Minot and William P. Murphy of Harvard and George H. Whipple of Rochester, honored for the discovery of the effect of liver in pernicious anemia; Edward A. Doisy of St. Louis for elucidating the chemistry of vitamin K; Sir Alexander Fleming of London and Sir Howard Florey and Ernst B. Chain of Oxford for the discovery and development of penicillin; Selman A. Waksman of Rutgers for the discovery of streptomycin; and Vincent duVigneaud of Cornell for the synthesis of hormones from the pituitary gland.

Of equal importance to drug therapy have been certain fundamental discoveries. For instance, John F. Enders, Frederick C. Robbins, and Thomas H. Weller received the Nobel Prize for growing poliomyelitis virus in tissue culture, which made possible the development of vaccines for poliomyelitis, measles, and rubella.

Independent institutes are represented by Nobel Prize winners such as Daniel Bovet of the Pasteur Institute, recognized for the synthesis of antihistamine drugs and muscle relaxants, and Philip S. Hench and Edward C. Kendall of the Mayo Clinic for their demonstration of the effectiveness of cortisone in arthritis. The most prominent of the independent institutes in America has been the Rockefeller Institute (now Rockefeller University), which has accentuated basic research, although it pioneered in the early decades of this century in making serums against pneumonia and meningitis. Research in universities is not only likely to be more consistently supported through good and bad weather; it is also the main training ground for future investigators. The pharmaceutical companies in the United States increased their scientific staffs for research and development from 11,400 in 1959 to 16,400 in 1965. Of these, 27 per cent had bachelor's degrees, 9 per cent master's degrees, and 23 per cent doctor's degrees. Most of those with doctoral degrees were trained in organic chemistry, medicine, biochemistry, pharmacology, or microbiology.[3] The universities must also train scientists in these fields for government, for private research institutes, and for their own teaching and research needs.

Government's support of medical research in modern times began when the public's imagination was captured by the discoveries of Pasteur. While the Pasteur Institute in France, founded to further these researches, was a private body, in Germany the first organized activities were financed by the government. It not only built a laboratory for Robert Koch, but later set up an institute for Paul Ehrlich, the father of chemotherapy for infections.[4] The Russian and Japanese governments also financed institutes for their leading bacteriologists.

In the United States, research on diphtheria antitoxin began in 1893 in the laboratories of the city of New York under Dr. William H. Park, who was to make this one of the outstanding bacteriological laboratories of the world.[5]

But the institution that was destined to be the biggest single force in American medical research began as a small laboratory in the Marine Hospital on Staten Island. Moved to Washington in 1902, it later became the Hygienic Laboratory; still later, the National Institute of Health; and eventually, the National Institutes of Health. It entered the field of drugs in 1902, when it was charged with the control of biologics, because it was then obliged to carry on research in serums and vaccines so as to set up standards for them.

Spurred by the need to establish standards, and by the practical problems posed by unsafe or ineffective vaccines and serums, investigators in the Hygienic Institute made a number of important discoveries. They found out how to eliminate tetanus as a complication of smallpox vaccination and devised a method for obtaining the maximum number of "takes," or successful vaccinations. They developed vaccines against Rocky Mountain spotted fever and typhus fever, and when it became clear that the human serum used in making yellow fever vaccine was sometimes transmitting the virus of serum hepatitis, they found out how to make a serum-free yellow fever vaccine.[6]

Government research on chemical drugs got under way more slowly. Although the Bureau of Chemistry of the Department of Agriculture opened a drug laboratory in 1903, the bureau's principal focus was foods until the second decade of the century. As a regulatory agency this bureau and its successor, the Food and Drug Administration, concentrated on methods of detecting and assaying drugs rather than developing new ones. Later the scientists in this agency began to study the actions of drugs in animals, but only in the last twenty years have they made a few tentative studies in human pharmacology.

The prevailing emphasis of the National Institutes of Health upon the infectious diseases began to shift in 1937, when the National Cancer Institute was created. Along with its studies on

the cause of cancer, this institute has maintained a strong interest
in the treatment of cancer with drugs. In 1955 it initiated a cancer
chemotherapy program "to find drugs that will cure cancer and
to make it possible for physicians to use them safely for the
control of all the malignant diseases."[7] It began with a budget of
about 1 million dollars a year, which had risen to 44 million dollars
by 1969.[8] This ambitious program is a co-ordinated effort of the
National Cancer Institute and of universities, industrial laboratories, and research institutes that are supported by grants and
contracts from the National Cancer Institute.

Other institutes with special programs for research in drugs
are the National Heart Institute and the National Institute of
Mental Health. The former is interested in drugs that lower the
level of fats in the blood and may prevent arteriosclerosis, drugs
for hypertension, drugs to treat heart failure and disturbances of
cardiac rhythm, and streptococcal vaccines for the prevention of
rheumatic fever. The National Institute of Mental Health is
supporting studies not only on the various drugs that stimulate or
depress the psyche, but also on the abuse of such drugs as the
narcotics, the barbiturates, the tranquilizers, and LSD (lysergic
acid diethylamide).

One of the newest institutes, the National Institute of General
Medical Sciences, is responsible for basic problems related to
disease and hence has assumed responsibility for the study of
the action of drugs at the cellular level, for the designing of drug
structures so as to produce certain therapeutic effects or to prevent certain adverse reactions, and for studies in the absorption,
metabolism, and excretion of drugs.[9] Recent work of the Division
of Biologics Standards will be considered in Chapter 10.

During World War II the United States was thrust into the
midst of the malaria problem. Quinine was unobtainable when
the Japanese occupied the East Indies, and the Germans held the
secrets of producing the antimalarial synthetics. The National
Research Council sponsored a many-pronged attack on the problem, which involved synthesizing hundreds of drugs and testing
them for their effect on malaria. Co-operating groups included
the army, the navy, the Public Health Service, the universities,

and the drug industry.[10] This research culminated in the discovery of chloroquine and the validation of its superior effect in the treatment of malaria. After the war the Army Research Institute continued the screening program for antimalarial compounds, and fortunately so, because in 1961 reports appeared of chloroquine-resistant cases of malaria caused by *Plasmodium falciparum* (the most virulent of the malarial parasites). At present, after screening over 80,000 compounds, investigators there are still looking for an ideal substitute for chloroquine.[11]

This brief account, though sketchy, shows that government agencies, acting alone or in concert with universities and the drug industry, have to their credit a number of significant achievements in research on drugs. They have confined their studies to the areas where the public health needs were the greatest, where the universities and the industrial laboratories were not moving fast enough to remedy obvious deficiencies, or where co-ordinated efforts appeared likely to be productive. They have consistently stayed out of the field of production when private companies were able to move in, but they have been ready and able to move into it quickly to fill a public need. This should be kept in mind especially when the responsiveness of the drug industry to the needs of the public is considered later on.

Research and development of drugs is only a small part of the function of universities and government; it is the major purpose of the pharmaceutical industry. Therefore, the evolution of this industry will be considered in detail.

Although drugs and drug mixtures have been prepared from earliest time, an industry capable of searching out and extracting drugs from nature on a wholesale scale, of synthesizing new chemical compounds, and of refashioning molecules had its beginnings only in the last decades of the nineteenth century. Around 1850 the era of heroic treatment by bleeding and purging had spent itself, and the nauseous mixtures of unappetizing herbs or animal excrements had largely disappeared from the practice of medicine, but there was very little to take their places. Mortal-

ity figures reflected this: the average age at death had changed
only slightly, from thirty-three years in the Middle Ages to forty
in the mid-nineteenth-century,[12] and this improvement could be
attributed almost entirely to advances in nutrition and sanitation.

As a result of their therapeutic impotence, physicians lost
face with the public, who were not impressed with the very real
gains that were being made in the sciences of physiology and
pathology. Even the benign Emerson attributed the doctor's help
mainly to "healthy talk, giving the right turn to the patient's
mind."[13] Partly as a result of planning and partly by chance, the
pharmaceutical industry moved in to fill the void in drug therapy.
Its success story is all the more striking because so little was there
before it began.

The first element in its success was the establishment of departments of pharmacology and bacteriology in the universities,
as already mentioned. Without these, the expertise necessary to
develop the processes of manufacture and control of quality, the
understanding of basic principles necessary to research, and the
recruits to work in the industrial laboratories would have been
lacking.

Another factor was the energy of a few apothecaries who, not
content with mixing prescriptions, set themselves the task of
making drugs available in wholesale quantities. Among the
earliest were Baumé in France some time before 1775, and
Fikentscher in Germany in 1788. The first factories set up exclusively for the production of drugs were probably Howard's in
England in 1807 and Trommsdorff's in Germany in 1813.[14] Riedel
started an apothecary shop in 1814, and Merck in 1816; in 1827
each began a wholesale business that soon became his whole
business. The newly discovered alkaloids, such as morphine,
quinine, and emetine, which were extracts from vegetable drugs,
opium, cinchona, and ipecac respectively, were an added
stimulus to wholesaling.

A third factor was the rise of the dye industry. Coal replaced
wood as an industrial fuel in England and on the Continent in
the seventeenth and eighteenth centuries, and gas was first made
from coal on a large scale in 1792. A by-product of this process

was coal tar, at first thought to be worthless but later found to have a number of uses, including the production of creosote. In 1856 William Henry Perkin, trying to synthesize quinine, produced instead aniline, a purple dye that was the first of a Pandora's box of aniline dyes. Thus was born the modern dye industry, which became in turn the mother of the pharmaceutical industry.

Although Perkin was an Englishman, the dye industry soon became concentrated mostly in Germany, because the German manufacturers, in contrast to the English, saw the need for basic research, and because the German universities were turning out enough young chemists to staff the research laboratories. Conditions were ripe for success in Switzerland also. The Geigy Company had been founded in 1758 for trade in and manufacture of spices, dyes, and drugs. It began to make synthetic dyes in the same year that Perkin discovered the process, and in 1859 another Swiss company, CIBA, Ltd., was founded for the same purpose.

The dye industry was highly competitive because as an appendage of the clothing industry it partook of the vagaries of taste and craving for novelty characteristic of the changing styles of clothing. The manufacturer had to keep inventing new colors, each of which was superseded in a short time by another. This required research laboratories, which in turn sought university-trained chemists.

Since dyes and drugs could both be synthesized from coal tar, the makers of dyes learned to use their laboratories and factories for the discovery and production of drugs also. Among the drugs first developed in this way were the salicylates, the barbiturates, and the analogues of cocaine. Later the dye and drug industries moved even closer together when Ehrlich showed that arsphenamine, structured in imitation of the azo group of dyes, would cure syphilis.

The development of the American drug industry can be traced through three periods, which I have called dependent, emergent, and dominant.

Until the nineteenth century the drugs used in America came almost entirely from England. The limited exceptions were a few herbs that had been taken over from Indian medicine and Glauber's and Epsom salts, which could be extracted locally.[15] The Revolutionary War had forced the new nation to make its own drugs or go without. The next fifty years saw a number of drug firms established. Some of the older, nationally known firms still in existence are Schieffelin & Co., founded in 1781, Wm. S. Merrell Co., in 1828, and McKesson & Robbins, Inc., in 1833. Others began during the period of industrialization around the Civil War, including Smith Kline & French Laboratories; E. R. Squibb & Sons; Wyeth Laboratories; Parke, Davis & Co.; Eli Lilly & Co.; and the Upjohn Company.[16]

These companies extracted the active principles from plants grown in America or imported from abroad, and improved the methods of making tablets, extracts, and mixtures more stable and palatable. Two of the leaders, Eli Lilly and Parke, Davis, made much of their profit by being "full line" drug houses; that is, by stocking all the drugs a physician would be called on to prescribe. But when it came to synthesizing drugs, this was done abroad; American companies either put the drug in medicinal form or merely sold the European product. Sometimes a company made an attractive preparation of a European discovery and popularized it in America, as the Upjohn Company did with phenolphthalein in Phenolax wafers.

When Koch, Pasteur, and their disciples demonstrated the possibilities of vaccines and serums, facilities for their manufacture were not available in this country. Dr. William H. Park, director of the laboratories of the New York City Health Department, sensing the need, built up over a number of years the country's foremost laboratory for the production of biologicals. But certain drug companies put pressure on him to stop selling his products, which were widely used because many doctors considered them superior to anything offered by commercial firms.[17] To produce diphtheria antitoxin by the improved methods he and others had devised, Dr. Park and Dr. Ernst Lederle, chief chemist in the New York City laboratory, formed the Lederle Antitoxin Laboratories and purchased a farm at Pearl River, New York. They, along with some of the established drug firms, developed diphtheria antitoxin and a number of vaccines that were equal or superior to anything manufactured abroad.

Toward the end of the dependent period the American market became so important that several European drug firms established branches in this country to sell their own products: Merck in 1899, Hoffman-LaRoche in 1905, and the Bayer and Burroughs-Wellcome companies in 1906.

World War I caught the American industry flat-footed. Germany had not only produced most of the synthetic drugs for the world market, but her firms had also kept secret the processes of manufacture. There was a mad scramble to learn to make them in America. Abbott Laboratories took up this work vigorously and by 1917 was producing barbital, the original barbiturate; procaine, a local anesthetic (known to most people by its trade name, Novocaine); and cinchophen, an effective drug for acute attacks of gout. At the same time the Dermatological Research Laboratories succeeded in making arsphenamine, Ehrlich's compound 606, the first effective specific for syphilis.[18]

Such experiences during the war stimulated the drug companies to continue increasing their facilities for research and production afterward. By 1920 the drug companies had set up forty-six research laboratories, and by 1940 research expenditures in several companies amounted to a half-million dollars a year or more. Whereas in 1880 there were 592 drug companies in the United States that produced 38 million dollars' worth of drugs a year, in 1940 before the onset of World War II there were nearly 1,100 plants and the annual value of their products was nearly 365 million dollars.[19]

But the German industry had not lain dormant, and its continuing productivity was matched by attempts to retain control. For instance, the American firm Sterling Products had purchased the U.S. branch of the Bayer Company from the United States government in 1918; yet it entered into an agreement with the German parent company, I. G. Farbenindustrie, whereby the latter bought half of the Winthrop Chemical Company (a subsidiary of Sterling Products), in return for which Winthrop obtained all of the German company's patents.[20]

World War II and the discovery of the sulfonamides were the stimuli that catapulted the American pharmaceutical industry into world leadership. Although the original sulfa drug was discovered in Germany, the method of its action explained by French investigators, and the first broadly acting sulfa drug, sulfapyridine, perfected in England, nevertheless the American pharmaceutical industry quickly developed its own analogues. Before long it was leading the world in production.

World War II spurred the production of drugs in this country by increasing the demand and by shutting off the supply from Germany and the countries it had seized. American industry could respond to the needs because it had developed technical and scientific competence since World War I. It pioneered especially in the discovery and development of vitamins and hormones and has done so more recently in other fields.

Interest and expertise in innovation in the field of serums, vaccines, and sulfonamides enabled the American drug industry to move rapidly into the antibiotic field. The first report of penicillin's effectiveness against human infections was made in 1940. In 1944 streptomycin was discovered at Rutgers and produced by Merck and Company in 1945. Chlortetracycline (Aureomycin) was discovered by scientists at Lederle Laboratories and marketed in 1948. Since then almost all of the innovation in antibiotics has occurred in the drug industry.[21]

In several other fields the first discoveries were made by foreign universities or drug companies, but the American industry moved in rapidly and made several modifications, some of which proved to have advantages over the original drugs. This was true for the barbiturates, the antihistaminics, and the oral antidiabetic drugs.

Which one of these groups—universities, government, or the drug industry—deserves the greatest credit for these new drugs? Some time ago an editorial appeared in the *American Journal of Public Health* entitled "Who Killed Cock Robin?"[22] which showed the absurdity of trying to distribute the kudos for advances in the health of the people. The threads of collective achievement cannot be disentangled; we cannot say that any one individual or group is responsible for the present-day chemotherapy of infectious diseases, or for the corticosteroids, or for the drugs that stimulate or depress the nervous system and the endocrine glands. What is more meaningful is the interrelationship and interdependence of the groups.

Penicillin was discovered in one university laboratory with the assistance of a grant from a private foundation and perfected in another university; then, under the stress of war, it was produced as a collaborative effort by twenty-two industrial firms in the United States under the sponsorship of the federal government, which provided subsidies. The program was spurred by the discovery in a research laboratory of the Department of Agriculture that corn steep liquor would increase the yield of the antibiotic one hundredfold and also that one of the strains of *Penicillium* from that laboratory would do a better job than those used before.[23] Who then is responsible for penicillin?

Although this collaboration occurred under the stress of war, it is by no means unique. The National Institute of Allergy and Infectious Diseases has programs for the development of vaccines against German measles, viruses that cause respiratory infections, and bacterial infections such as pneumonia and meningitis. Some of the work is done in the institute, but the major part is done under contract by drug companies and universities.[24] The National Cancer Institute has supported the search for anticancer drugs and their investigation in animals and man; this program is carried on both at the institute and at institute-subsidized universities and drug companies.[25] In all, various federal agencies spent over 100 million dollars on drug-related research in 1968,[26] as compared with 521 million dollars spent for research and development by the seventy-eight research-oriented firms in the Pharmaceutical Manufacturers Association.[27]

An even more important reason why credit for discoveries cannot be attributed to any one group is the fact that every discovery of a new drug today must be based upon other knowledge, both in the basic and clinical sciences. Though the credit may go to a single investigator, it really belongs to an army of laboratory and clinical scientists, practicing physicians, technicians, nurses, and others. None could produce today's new drugs by himself; all can do the job together.

If the credit cannot be parceled out with exactitude, the assignment of responsibility often can be. Because industrial firms seek profits and the unversities seek knowledge, the former accentuate applied, and the latter, basic, research. However, in recent years the larger pharmaceutical firms have encouraged basic research, too, because they believe that in the long run it will pay off in dollars. In 1962 the drug industry spent for basic research 16.3 per cent of the 203.5 million dollars budgeted for research conducted in their own plants as compared with an average of 4 per cent for all industry.[28]

On the other hand, since true scientific investigation means pursuing any problem that interests the investigator, university scientists sometimes do applied research. Doctors are particularly interested in getting sick people well and in preventing illness. Consequently, much applied research is carried out in medical schools and hospitals.

Governments are service-motivated and tend to foster research establishments that will manifestly benefit public health, but the federal government has found that basic research is necessary to push forward the nation's capacity for applied research, especially in areas that are not receiving enough attention; they have also come to realize, as has industry, that to recruit and retain good scientists they must allow them to pursue their own research interests part of the time—and this often means basic research. Thus all three groups pursue both basic and applied research, although the emphasis differs.

The contention of the Pharmaceutical Manufacturers Association is that "the primary role of government in medical research is to encourage the expansion and enrichment of the flow of fundamental knowledge, sometimes referred to as basic research," leaving "the discovery and design of new medicines" to the pharmaceutical industry.[29] Aside from the reasons already given why this sharp division cannot be made, an additional factor is that such a separation of responsibility enables the drug industry to claim patent monopolies and the profits that they reap. Yet the discovery and design of a drug are almost always built upon basic research that has gone before, and the application of the drug to disease depends upon knowledge of disease processes and how to diagnose them. Should the chap who made the icing for the cake take the whole cake home? This problem will be discussed further when we consider the economics of the drug industry.

The Lord hath created medicines out of the earth;
and he that is wise will not abhor them.
Of such doth the apothecary make a confection;
and of his works there is no end;
and from him is peace over all the earth.

—ECCLESIASTICUS 38:3–8

3

The Production and Laboratory Testing of Drugs

After a drug is found in nature or invented in a laboratory, an efficient method must be devised for producing it in large quantities, and it must be subjected to rigid tests in the laboratory. Finally, ethical considerations demand that it be thoroughly studied in animals before being given to patients. Although manufacturing and testing are distinct operations, they are considered together in this chapter because they are both carried out mainly in industrial plants and because they often take place simultaneously.

". . . The innovator who develops a commercial product or process and tries it in the marketplace contributes as much or more to technological innovation and economic growth than the originator of the idea," says Harvey Brooks, dean of Harvard's School of Engineering.[1] Although most people might not minimize the role of the man with the original idea as much as Dean Brooks does, everyone would agree on the importance and necessity of producing quantities of sufficiently pure, consistently potent replicas of drugs that have heretofore only been prepared in the research laboratory. The early development of penicillin was cited in Chapter 2 as an instance where the government encouraged and supported and industry produced. For even after Florey and his team of investigators had saved several lives with the tiny quantities of penicillin they had been able to make in their laboratory, British pharmaceutical companies did not try to manufacture it because these firms were swamped with work in the midst of a world war. American manufacturers, stimulated by grants from the Office of Scientific Research and Development, took up the task.[2] In a few years penicillin production rose from zero in 1942 to 21 billion units in 1943, to 1,633 billion units in 1944, and continued to soar to reach 1,202 trillion units in 1964.[3] The cost of production dropped concomitantly so that in the past two decades it has cost less to make a dose of penicillin than to make the ampule in which it is sealed. This is but one example of hundreds in which ingenuity, drive, and practical skills have moved American industry into a position of leadership in a developing technology.

But the move from laboratory to factory is not without hazards. Thus, the president of Merck & Co., Inc., complained that in the early attempts to produce cortisone "a key reaction (one chemical step in thirty-five) which worked well in the laboratory failed when it was expanded in size to meet production requirements."[4] To make the transition smoother, most drugs are produced in a pilot plant, where the differences between the research laboratory and the factory can be detected before mass production is begun. This step adds time and expense but prevents costly, large-scale failures.

After the pilot plant comes production in quantity. It is here that manufacturing on a large scale proves its efficiency and often forces smaller firms to buy in bulk because they cannot compete economically with the large companies. Thus a drug may be manufactured by only one or two companies while it is placed in its final form as a tablet, capsule, or solution by a dozen or more different firms.

Pharmaceutical preparations made from the same chemical may vary greatly in palatability, keeping qualities, and absorbability. Meeting the problems raised by these requirements and assuring uniformity in these areas often call for a great deal of ingenuity, industry, and money. For years after its value had been proved, penicillin could not be given orally, partly because large quantities were needed and the antibiotic was in short supply and partly because it was inactivated by the gastric juice. Eventually, when tablets were devised that contained adequate alkali buffers, the oral method became overnight the cheapest, most convenient, and most widely used method of administration.

In recent years a whole new class of "delayed absorption" preparations have been invading the drug market. By coating particles or layers of the drug with substances that dissolve slowly in the intestinal juices, the pharmaceutical companies have devised preparations that extend absorption over several hours. Such preparations are convenient for patients, especially for nighttime medication and for forgetful businessmen during the day. Unfortunately, the drug companies saw the sales potential of these formulations before they solved the problems of absorption from the intestines.[5] Thus, preparations for delayed absorption sometimes smack more of gimmickry than of science. Now, under the stern and vigilant eyes of the FDA (Food and Drug Administration), the drug companies are retracing their steps and looking for more solid facts upon which to base their processes and their claims.

Finally, the modern pharmaceutical preparations are devised to flag doctors' and patients' attention by distinctive shapes, vivid colors, pleasant tastes, and attractive packaging. Lilies are gilded here as in other industries, but in the drug industry, because of regulation by the federal government, we can be sure that the product is a good one, gilded or not.

A characteristic feature of manufacturing drugs is "quality control." Because small variations in the quantity or quality of a drug can mean the difference between sickness and health or even between life and death, careful checks must be made on the uniformity and purity of finished drugs. A difference of as little as one milligram of an intravenous preparation of certain digitalis derivatives can cause the death of a patient who has previously received digitalis. Another example is the contamination of other drugs by penicillin. In the year beginning July 1, 1964, over two hundred drug products were recalled after they had been placed on the market, and of these, ninety were recalled because they were contaminated by this common antibiotic.[6] Since approximately one person in forty is hypersensitive to penicillin and since as small a dose as one tablet taken by mouth has caused death in highly sensitive persons, this record cannot be lightly brushed aside.

It has been claimed that ". . . no other industry is so dependent on the infallibility of its end product as the pharmaceutical industry. . . . While a manufacturer of defective piston rings has another chance, the distribution of a contaminated drug spells ruin."[7] For this reason quality control is usually separated from the manufacturing division, and in a properly run company, the head of quality control not only reports directly to top management but has the final say on the acceptance or rejection of any batch of a drug. This insures that the control system, as Earle Meyers of the FDA said, will "observe the regular and continuous use of all reasonable methods, procedures and operations that are necessary to ensure the uniformity of pharmaceutical products as to safety, and effectiveness, including the use of those which will minimize the human, mechanical, and other errors throughout all phases of production and assure the user that his package of the product has all the characteristics of identity, strength, quality which it is represented or purported to possess."[8]

Production and quality control cost money, but the American pharmaceutical industry with its vast resources is adequate to the task. In the drug industry as a whole the number of employees engaged in quality control is about 20 per cent of all personnel involved in production.[9] *Drug Trade News* reported that in 1965 the drug manufacturers on whom it was able to obtain information spent 32.9 per cent of their sales dollar on manufacturing.[10] Some idea of the size of these expenditures can be obtained from the amounts spent for this purpose by individual companies during that year: Abbott Laboratories, over 98 million dollars; Parke, Davis & Company, nearly 82 million dollars; and Upjohn Company, nearly 66 million dollars. The ability of the pharmaceutical industry to shoulder these tasks was pointed up by the anonymous author of *Facts About Pharmacy and Pharmaceuticals*, who claimed: "Had some nineteenth-century Sir Alexander Fleming discovered penicillin, industry would have been in the same powerless position as a Renaissance workshop faced with the problem of building airplanes from the plans of Leonardo da Vinci."[11]

As a matter of fact, the pharmaceutical industry was in exactly that position at the end of the nineteenth century, when the French and German bacteriologists had produced diphtheria antitoxin. As mentioned previously, American laboratories were unable to make this serum properly and in sufficient quantities, and the New York City Health Laboratory produced it not only for use in New York City but for sale elsewhere.[12] Today, the financial and technical strength of the leading American pharmaceutical manufacturers assures their ability to move into the production of any drug as rapidly as government laboratories, if not more rapidly. Only when commercial firms are unwilling to act, because they do not see the prospect of sufficient profits, must the government take the initiative.

In addition to money, it takes time to set up the procedures and the apparatus for the manufacture and quality control of a new drug, so that several months to a year may often be required. Fortunately, other things are going on at the same time. The first of these is the testing of the drugs in animals.

In our society today it is generally accepted that a drug should be tested in the lower animals before it is given to man. The concept that men's lives are more precious than those of the lower animals has been built into our ethics over thousands of years. "If anything is sacred," said Walt Whitman, "the human body is sacred."

If animals are to be man's surrogate in drug testing, how good a substitute are they? Most of the techniques employed in screening drugs in animals were developed to guide the chemist in synthesizing new drugs.[13] Thus the techniques are not necessarily suited to detecting toxic reactions. To make them serve as red lights for clinical testing, it seems obvious that the results of tests in the lower animals and man must be compared. Yet only in recent years have any systematic studies of this kind been made.

In a study of sixteen different kinds of adverse drug effects, it was found that animals were altogether useless in predicting nine.[14] When tests on drugs in rats, dogs, and humans were compared, 49 per cent of the predictions that abnormal physical signs would occur in man derived from studies in rats, and 55 per cent from studies in dogs were confirmed in man.[15] Even when the tests on rats and dogs were combined, only 68 per cent of the signs observed in either of the animal species were verified in man. The absence of abnormal physical signs was correctly predicted in 79 per cent of cases, giving an overall score of 74 per cent for the two animal species.[16] To put it the other way, one fourth of the physical signs that occurred in man after the use of certain drugs could not be predicted by the tests with these two species of animal. Among 41 adverse reactions most often observed in 11,115 patients treated with 77 different drugs or combinations of drugs, 22 could not be satisfactorily tested in the lower animals.[17]

Furthermore, although the science of pharmacology is over a hundred years old, the animals used today are not necessarily chosen on a scientific basis. Mice, rats, guinea pigs, and rabbits are easily bred, easily handled, and therefore relatively cheap. Dogs and cats are handy and familiar. Thus these animals are the ones commonly used. Tests in other animals such as monkeys, chimpanzees, and pigs have been used less extensively.

Certain animals are particularly valuable for studying particular classes of drugs. Many infections in the subhuman primates, for instance, resemble those of humans. The first experimental transmission of mumps, measles, and infectious mononucleosis was accomplished in monkeys. Syphilis was first successfully transmitted to a chimpanzee. The virulence of the different strains of dengue, West Nile fever, yellow fever, and poliomyelitis viruses has long been observed to be similar in man and monkey. Recently the mysterious neurological disease kuru was shown to be a "slow virus" disease by inoculation into chimpanzees. Anthrax, plague, pneumococcic pneumonia, and the common cold have similar characteristics in monkeys and in humans. And growing polio viruses in monkey-kidney tissue culture led to the first successful polio vaccine. Thus studies of infections and the effects of drugs on infections are fertile fields for research on primates.

Yet just because the lower primates are closest to man in the path of evolution does not mean that they ingest, metabolize, and excrete every drug as man does. These processes must be studied for each class of drugs in each species of animal. Morphine, for instance, has a depressing effect upon dogs and rats as it does in man, while it stimulates cats, goats, and horses. On the other hand, a narcotic that is sometimes used in man in place of morphine, meperidine, is broken down so rapidly in the dog that it has little effect.[18] Therefore, when a drug is being tested that is like others previously studied, the animals selected for testing are those that most resemble man in their reactions to the drug's analogues. But when a drug without previously tested analogues is being studied, the animals used for testing may or may not be relevant, and it is important that pharmacological studies be started in man as soon as possible to find out which of the lower animals most resemble his reactions. Extensive studies can then be made on those animals.

When many different species are explored, for each drug one or more animals will be found to resemble humans in the way they metabolize the drug or in the adverse reactions that they exhibit when the drug is given them. Up to now, this ideal situation exists for only a few drugs. Only careful studies of the animal traditionally used for each class of drugs, and other animals as well, will fill in the blank spaces. Until these are filled in, we shall undoubtedly have to continue the practice—wasteful of time and money—of giving a new drug to certain animals because this has become a routine practice.

At present, tests for toxicity are designed to determine the maximum dose that is tolerated safely, the nature of toxic symptoms, signs, and tissue changes that will appear when still higher doses are given, and the effects of long-term administration (taking into consideration how long the drug will be given to patients).

The acute experiments (lasting for a few days to a few weeks) are usually done on several species, such as mice, rats, guinea pigs, and dogs. The subacute studies (lasting approximately three months) and the chronic studies (requiring up to a year or more) are usually done on two species, such as rats and dogs. Special studies are made of the changes in the blood cells, the serum enzymes, tests for the function of the liver and kidney, pathologic changes in the organs of animals that have died or are sacrificed, and the effects of the drug upon the fetus in pregnant animals.[19]

A drug found acceptable under these standards will probably be safe in humans. Yet no thoughtful investigator is satisfied with the tests at his disposal at present. We need better techniques for determining the physiological changes in animals receiving drugs and more research on the factors causing malignancies, hypersensitivity phenomena, fetal abnormalities, and the destruction of the blood cells in animals, and their relationship to similar phenomena in man.[19] We need more correlations between the findings in animals and man to see which animals and which tests are most revealing.

These facts have a bearing on the FDA regulations regarding the numbers and varieties of animals that must be studied before a new drug can be given to man, but before we consider regulation by government agencies of the efficacy and toxicity of drugs, we must first look at the evaluation of drugs in humans and then at the economic factors that relate to the discovery, production, and laboratory testing of drugs.

They [physicians] learne their skill by endangering
our lives; and to make proof and experiments
of their medicines, they care not to kill us.
—PLINY THE ELDER (A.D. 23–79)

The investigator, engaged in clinical research,
has always been concerned about the safety of
his subjects. . . . Frequently, however, he must
ultimately experience the feeling of loneliness
which accompanies the exploration of new areas,
without the benefit of past experience from
any source, and with only scientific knowledge,
integrity, and a deep-seated conscience as a guide.
—DR. AUSTIN SMITH

4

The Evaluation
of Drugs in Humans

After drugs are tested in the laboratory and in animals, another important step must be taken before they can be used extensively in patients: they have to be studied in man to see whether they are safe and effective, to see how they work and whether they can be made to work better. Whereas the past half century saw the development of a science and technology for the testing of drugs in animals, the evaluation of drugs in humans did not receive much attention until the past few years. Now rather suddenly many people in the medical profession, in the drug industry, and in the government have become interested, and they find the methods inadequate and the human problems unsettled. Yet move into this field we must, because the test in man is the ultimate test, of vital importance to anyone who takes a dose of a drug—which means everyone at some time or other.

Some studies of drugs are directed to determining safety, some to determining efficacy, and others to finding out how a drug works and under what conditions, but as often as possible observations are made on all of these at one time. Efficacy is important because, as we have seen in the chapter on the discovery of drugs, doctors at times have used measures that were completely worthless or at least worthless against the diseases for which they were prescribed. For instance, reasoning falsely by analogy, doctors were deluded into using quinine, which was highly effective against malaria, for other fevers on which it hadn't the slightest effect. In conformity with the best practice of the time George Washington was bled and blistered, poulticed and purged, in an attempt to cure the throat infection that took his life.[1] Examples of ineffective drugs can be found today. When guinea pigs are deficient in bioflavinoids, which are substances extracted from citrus fruits, the walls of their capillary blood vessels are abnormally permeable. On these shaky grounds, bioflavinoids have been promoted for a variety of human ills: diseases of the blood vessels, diabetes, allergies, various types of hemorrhage, and the common cold. The National Research Council disagreed; it recently concluded that bioflavinoids have no therapeutic effect in man. As a result, the FDA moved to prevent their sponsors from making such a claim.[2] If the FDA succeeds, it will in effect remove these drugs from the market—for who would buy a drug for which no therapeutic effect can be claimed?

Knowing how a drug is absorbed, combined with body fluids, metabolized, and excreted is important because it will help the physician achieve better therapeutic effects, prevent adverse reactions, arrange the doses more efficiently, and perhaps more important still, help the investigator find analogues of the drug that would act differently in the body and thus be more suitable for therapy. A knowledge of how the drug acts is important because it will lead us to the optimal doses, methods of administration, spacing of doses, duration of therapy, and prevention of side effects, and will tell the physician how to judge when the drug is doing the most good for his patient.

Most important of all, we have to be sure that the drugs we take are as safe as possible. Every drug has at some time in some person caused an adverse reaction (an unfavorable effect apart from the drug's intended therapeutic action, varying in severity from slight headache, dizziness, or nausea all the way to high fever, shock, or death). But some drugs cause toxic effects in a high proportion of persons. Yet they must be used because the disease they combat is serious and no better therapy is available. This is true, for instance, of most of the anticancer drugs. In a less serious disease, however, it is better to do without the potentially unsafe drug altogether. To use a highly toxic drug for the common cold, for instance, would be unthinkable. Also, substitute drugs are often available for a relatively unsafe drug so that its elimination is a gain in safety and no loss in over-all therapy.

Some adverse effects are discovered when the first tests are made; others are not detected for months or years. Dinitrophenol, a drug that was used to reduce weight, was apparently not toxic in animals nor did it appear harmful in the first tests in man. Only after it had been used extensively in humans was it found to produce cataracts. The oral contraceptive drugs apparently increase the propensity for blood clotting in some persons but in so few that the drugs had been used widely by thousands of women for more than three years before the first suspicions of this effect were reported in the medical literature.[3]

Although the last word on the adverse reactions to a drug may not be in for years—we are still adding to our knowledge on the toxic effects of digitalis—most reactions are detected early. We might liken the process to passage through a series of sieves. The animal tests, the first sieve, screen out the great majority of adverse reactions; then the preliminary tests in man, like a sieve with smaller pores, screen out some more; and lastly, the finest sieve of all is the use of the drug in large numbers of persons. This final sieve can detect a reaction such as agranulocytosis (the disappearance of the white blood cells from the blood, greatly increasing susceptibility to infection) from aminopyrine, which is estimated to occur in one out of fifty thousand persons who receive this drug. By the proper use of the techniques available to us today and by continually searching to improve the methods, we can have confidence that the drugs we take will produce a minimum of adverse reactions.

Sometimes an adverse reaction affects only particular persons. Thalidomide was relatively nontoxic for most people, but it caused pregnant women to have babies with seal-like flippers instead of arms or with no arms at all. (See p. 200.) Chloramphenicol is destroyed efficiently by the older child and adult but not by the newborn, a fact that was not detected until some newborn babies who were receiving chloramphenicol went into shock because the drug accumulated in their blood.

Not all drugs producing adverse effects come to a bad end. When the first antihistamines were used for hay fever, they were found to cause drowsiness. Laboratory scientists rushed to develop analogues that would have less of this side effect. Some were produced, but along with these, other analogues were found that had *more* of this side effect, and the latter were marketed as drugs to induce sleep.

It must be emphasized that no drug is or can be made completely safe. Even the commonest drug, aspirin, will occasionally cause bleeding from the stomach and in large doses will always cause ringing in the ears. The simple alkaline salts, used for heartburn and stomach discomforts and the treatment of ulcers of the stomach and duodenum, if taken in excess, can tax the body's facilities for getting rid of excess calcium, which is then deposited in various organs where it may do harm. Yet if we cannot achieve complete safety, we can come close to it by eliminating the more toxic drugs among those having the same therapeutic effect, by excluding highly toxic drugs (except for the treatment of life-threatening diseases such as cancer), and by learning all we can about adverse reactions and disseminating that information to doctors. Our aim would be to prevent adverse reactions wherever possible and to detect them early and treat them properly if they do occur.

The clinical evaluation of drugs has been divided into three phases:

PHASE 1. This represents the first tests in man, which are primarily directed toward finding gross or obvious toxic effects and determining how the drug is absorbed, metabolized, and eliminated and how it affects certain physiologic functions, such as blood pressure, heart rate, etc. These tests are usually done in healthy volunteers; sometimes, as in the case of anticancer drugs, they are given first to patients who have the disease they are designed to treat.

PHASE 2. In this phase a limited number of patients are treated with the drug and observed for the effect of the drug on the prevention or control of a disease or the improvement of symptoms, although adverse effects and physiologic reactions are noted along the way.

PHASE 3. The purpose of this phase is to establish the effectiveness, safety, and optimal dosage of the drug for the diseases against which it may be useful. To accomplish these objectives, larger numbers of patients must be treated—sometimes very large numbers. This is particularly true when the drug is intended for prophylaxis. For instance, studies on the effectiveness of the continuous administration of isoniazid in preventing tuberculosis in persons who had been intimately exposed to this disease involved 69,318 persons by 1963,[4] and more have been added since. A more publicized experiment, the large-scale trials of killed poliomyelitis vaccine in 1954, involved 1,829,916 children.[5]

These three phases of testing are required by the federal government before a drug may be marketed in this country, but it has been suggested that the initial period after the drug is available for sale be labeled Phase 4, since new uses or unknown adverse reactions are frequently discovered after the doctors in practice begin to use it. It is to be expected that the increased surveillance by the FDA under the Drug Amendments Act of 1962 will detect more adverse reactions before drugs are released for sale than in the past, but it is a vain hope that we can detect them all. Some reactions are too infrequent or too subtle for the smaller number of preliminary tests to ferret them all out. Thus we must depend upon practicing physicians to detect adverse reactions. How to achieve better reporting will be discussed in later chapters.

The study of drugs in humans, called clinical pharmacology, is but one part of the larger discipline of clinical investigation and uses the same tools. Laboratory investigation uses exact methods, a definite quantity of a chemical in a test tube, accurately calibrated apparatus to count radioactive emissions, etc. Clinical investigation may be rigorously exact at times; at other times it depends on such uncertain evidence as the patient's recital of his symptoms, or upon the effect of a drug in a patient who is already reacting abnormally because he is sick. Testing drugs for relief of headache is an example of the former, and the use of drugs to bring a patient out of shock following a serious automobile accident is an example of the latter. Moreover, the human subject may be affected emotionally because he is being observed, and this in turn may affect the measurements being made.

All of the tools for diagnosing sick people are used in clinical investigation when they are relevant: history-taking and physical examination; observations of the structure and actions of organs by the X-ray or electrocardiograph; placing tubes in the stomach, bladder, or heart; examination of body fluids and excreta, such as blood, cerebrospinal fluid, urine, or feces; biopsy of pieces of organs and tissues; and finally, the autopsy when the end result is death. To these tools others have been added. The clinical investigator may ask his patients to walk on a treadmill, harnessed with wires attached to an electrocardiograph, to measure the effect of propanolol, a new drug that relieves the pain of angina pectoris. He may even induce an infection, such as the common cold, to look for its cause or to find a drug that will cure it. Thus clinical investigation is more varied and at the same time more difficult than laboratory investigation. Investigators must continually strive to make it as exact as possible.

Let us look at some of the matters with which clinical investigation must be concerned, especially as it applies to the evaluation of drugs.

To whom should a drug be given in order to try it? This depends on the nature of the drug, the severity of the disease being treated or prevented, and the phase of the investigation. The initial tests of a potentially dangerous drug to combat cancer would be justified only in cancer patients, whereas a remedy for the common cold might be tested with impunity in normal subjects. And of course if a new drug has already been given to a number of persons without ill effects, it can then be given to a wider spectrum of people.

In the past it was not uncommon for new drugs to be given to members of various "out groups," the inmates of charity institutions, the sick poor on hospital wards, members of disadvantaged races, and criminals. In a throwback to barbarism, the Nazis even subjected political prisoners to crippling and fatal experiments. As I have shown elsewhere,[6] present-day ethics do not tolerate experiments performed on persons who are not in a position to give intelligent, informed, and wholehearted consent. This means that investigators cannot draw subjects at will from the reservoir of charity patients as before. Moreover, this reservoir is shrinking as the charity patient disappears. As a result, present-day clinical investigators are working more intensively with four groups and are turning also to a fifth.

First, as the educational level of the population rises, people understand the need to test drugs properly; thus, many patients will co-operate when the object of an experiment is explained to them. Second, some well persons, students for instance, are willing to be experimental subjects to earn extra money. A third group, conscientious objectors to military service, offer themselves as experimental subjects because they believe this is one of the noblest sacrifices they can make. Prisoners form a fourth group. Today's ethics require not only the voluntary consent of a prisoner but also that the rewards offered not be so great as to impel him to submit to experiments of which he would not otherwise approve. Working within the framework of such ethical codes, investigators have increased progressively the amount of drug testing done in penitentiaries, and some pharmaceutical companies have actually financed buildings adjacent to penitentiaries for this purpose. This appears to be a salutary movement, since such tests not only benefit society but also give a prisoner an opportunity to redeem himself in his own eyes and in the eyes of others.[7]

However, prisoners when used as experimental subjects are an ever-present temptation to exploitation. The public was recently shocked by allegations that when drugs were tested in Alabama prisons the prisoners were not told of the possible effects of the tests, and were not always examined thoroughly beforehand, watched carefully during the experiments, nor treated properly when reactions occurred. A committee of the Alabama Medical Society reported that, although useful and practical contributions had been made by the staff and the President, Dr. Austin R. Stough, of Southern Food and Drug Research, which had been operating a program of research in Alabama prisons for several years, many deficiencies existed, which constituted hazards to the health of the prisoners tested. These included an inadequately trained staff, insufficient interest in the prisoner as a patient, lack of medical supervision, unsatisfactory conditions for treatment of prisoners, the lack of prior review of the tests by professional peers, and overcrowding of facilities because too many tests were undertaken at one time.[8] Recommendations will be made in this chapter which, if followed, will act as safeguards against deficiencies such as these.

The fifth source of drug testing today is more questionable: the testing of drugs in other countries where the standards of consent may not be so rigorously applied. This trend has caused a number of drug companies to test and market drugs abroad before placing them on the American market.

When a doctor prescribes a well-known drug for a patient, it is assumed that he knows what he is doing, and the patient's consent is therefore implied. But administering an untried drug is different; it is research, and the distinction has been well stated in a recent conference sponsored by the American College of Cardiology:

> . . . *in practice, the patient seeks the doctor; in research specific patients are sought and selected. In practice, diagnosis, treatment, and care are provided for the specific condition as long as needed; in research, treatment lasts only during the period of investigation. It sometimes terminates before improvement and sometimes continues for after-study. In practice, the patient pays the doctor, whereas study patients or subjects are often paid or given care in exchange. But most importantly, practice is limited to the accepted modes, whereas the experimental study usually involves the untested and untried.*
>
> *The patient-subject's role correspondingly differs. As a patient, he is expected to recognize his illness or possible illness and follow generally understood instructions. The subject, on the other hand, is held, almost on contractual terms, to follow study requirements. For good reason he may leave the study, but his role is that of a partner.*[9]

Out of the guilt engendered by previous misdeeds has arisen a set of ethical rules that, although not unanimously agreed upon in every detail, contain a central core of concurrence. These rules are well stated in the Declaration of Helsinki, adopted by the World Medical Association in 1964 and subsequently endorsed by the major medical societies in this country and abroad. It is a recognition that "the patient, however humble and however ill, in whatever degree derelict and forlorn, has sacred rights which the physician must always put ahead of his burning curiosity."[10]

Central to the proper protection of the person experimented upon is his agreement. The consent of the patient or subject to whom a new drug is given is not implied and therefore must be explicit, specific, and based on an understanding by the subject of the risks involved. Although many people believe consent should be in writing because this helps to prove that it was actually obtained, this is not necessary, provided that the subject gives explicit consent orally, in which case a witness is always desirable. Nor is the subject's signature accepted as *prima facie* evidence that he gave his full and free and understanding consent. To understand, the subject must have received an explanation of what is to be done and the risks that might reasonably be anticipated, couched in language he can comprehend. Whether another responsible person can legally give consent for a minor or for a mentally incompetent subject is a disputed question; if not, it is difficult to see how we can ever establish the safety of any new drug for children or know what doses to give.

Many protests have been heard against the FDA regulations requiring informed consent. (See Chapter 11.) Some contend that the risks of taking a new drug are not known and therefore cannot be explained, and that even the known risks cannot be explained to the uneducated and the unintelligent. These objections contain a modicum of truth, but an experimental subject should expect an explanation of the hazards as the experimenter understands them. If the investigator is up on his subject, as he should be, the law can hardly ask for more than that. As for the uneducated, the explanation can be put in terms he will understand. The subject whose intelligence is so low that he cannot comprehend any explanation had better be omitted from hazardous experiments.[11]

When the subject is also a patient and the new drug is given because it may benefit him, his consent is still necessary, although the explanation of why it is given and its hazards may be limited or omitted if the explanation is likely to be more harmful to the patient than the experiment, as in the case of a drug given for cancer when the patient has not been told the nature of his illness. But even here it is wise for the physician to take a responsible relative into his confidence.

The physician treating a patient rather than a volunteer subject is in a delicate position. He is the patient's doctor, to whom the patient has relinquished the responsibility to use whatever measures are in the patient's best interest. On the other hand, he is experimenting, with the aim of advancing science, and this objective may run counter to the patient's comfort and safety. The physician's safest course is to explain to the patient-subject what he is doing (or to some responsible relative or friend if a full explanation might cause undue anxiety in the patient). He should also share his responsibility with colleagues by requesting a consultation, by seeking the approval of a committee of peers, or by having the patient cared for by another physician who would pass upon the propriety of investigations.

Approval of human experimentation by committees of peers seems to me to be the best method for most circumstances. Although this had been the practice in a few hospitals for years, it was forced on others by an epoch-making directive from the National Institutes of Health. This required, in effect, that grantee-institutions establish committees to pass on the propriety of all experiments conducted on human subjects.[12] Although such committees do consume time, can cause delays, and occasionally may even block worth-while research, on the positive side they can help by improving the design of the experiment, by curbing excessive zeal in investigators, and especially by protecting the careful, conscientious investigator. Active committees of this kind in every hospital, listened to by investigators and backed up by senior staff members and administrators, would go a long way toward assuring the proper protection of subjects of human experiments. Experiments conducted outside of hospitals could be conducted under the sponsorship of committees appointed by the county medical society.

Unfortunately, investigating the hazards of new drugs is a hazard to the investigator, too.

> *. . . Twentieth century medical research is forced to*
> *exist in the legal climate of the eighteenth century.*
> *. . . [T]he courts have used the term "experimentation"*
> *in the sense of malpractice. . . . The situation of*
> *the controlled clinical trial, for instance, has not*
> *yet been litigated. Consequently, no judicial forum*
> *has squarely faced the significant difference between*
> *(a) scientifically developed deviation from*
> *established practice, embodying careful regulation*
> *of conditions toward comprehension of new*
> *medical principles and (b) changes introduced by*
> *a practitioner through lack of skill, negligence, or*
> *intent, but without prior demonstration of research.*[13]

To give proper protection to the investigator of new drugs and to the subjects used, the sponsor should provide the cost of liability insurance whenever a new drug is being tested. This should be a consistent and expected procedure, and its cost should be included as a matter of course in the expenses of such tests.

More important than this, the necessity of investigating new drugs and the procedures required for such investigations should be recognized in the statutes. It would be advisable if the concept of "liability without fault" could be utilized, whereby injury to an experimental subject could be recognized and compensated for when he was harmed, even though there was no evidence of a mistake or omission on the part of the investigator. Clinical investigation has come of age; it is time the law recognizes it.

Who is qualified to study the effects of drugs in humans? Certainly not every doctor. Most investigations require a detailed knowledge of the actions of drugs; extensive experience with the diseases for which treatment is being tried; special techniques that will measure efficacy, detect adverse reactions, and trace the metabolic fate of drugs; and special facilities for the care of patients and laboratory testing to make these things possible. Many physicians do not have such special skills and knowledge.

They do not have access to special facilities, nor have they been trained to devise the kinds of experiments that will yield valid results. It follows, then, that the initial experiments must be carried out by someone who is familiar with such studies.

Opinions are divided as to whether drugs are best studied by a doctor grounded in pharmacology who learns how to use drugs in humans, called a clinical pharmacologist, or by a doctor skilled in research in a specialty of clinical medicine, a clinical investigator, who learns enough pharmacology to do the job. But, as I have shown elsewhere, the need for different approaches to the study of drugs and the scarcity of doctors with proper qualifications and facilities mean that doctors in both groups should be encouraged to make such studies.[14]

When preliminary studies have been done and the drug must be tried in much larger numbers of patients, clinicians with less experience in research can participate profitably. Expertise in devising rigidly controlled experiments can be provided by others when necessary. Several excellent controlled clinical trials have been conducted in which a central planning group devised the experiment, sent the drugs out under code names, collected the data, and tabulated them. The practicing physician administered the drug (without knowing which patient was receiving a particular drug) and made the necessary observations and laboratory tests on the patients. Examples are the studies on isoniazid in the prevention of tuberculosis conducted in many hospitals throughout the United States under the sponsorship of the Public Health Service[15] and the collaborative studies of the College of General Practitioners in England.[16]

In a time when physicians of all kinds are scarce, the pharmaceutical companies sometimes feel that they are holding out a beggar's bowl at the very bottom of the line. The reasons are that only a small fraction of all doctors are interested in investigation, fewer still in studies on drugs, and most of these more interested in basic studies on the action of drugs than studies in patients. The drug companies meet the problem in various ways: by doing many of their tests abroad, by contracting with physicians who make a business of testing drugs, by bringing testing facilities under their own control, and by helping younger physicians learn the methods of clinical pharmacology. Of course they realize, as does everyone else, that in the long run it will be necessary for medical schools to train more physicians in these techniques. (This will be discussed further in Chapter 13.)

Some of the larger companies have followed the example of Eli Lilly & Co. by establishing or supporting facilities in which physicians employed by them can test drugs in patients or in normal subjects. If these facilities are associated with a medical school, so as to assure both consistency in scientific standards and freedom from charges of bias, this method works well.

In the face of stiff competition for the few investigators closely connected with medical schools, some of the smaller companies have deliberately sought younger physicians who have hospital facilities and who have an interest in, but no training in, clinical investigation. The company's director of clinical investigation and his staff help these doctors design their experiments and advise them on the treatment of the data. This system can be valuable in overcoming the present shortage of investigators, but it has obvious hazards. So long as the guidance is limited to advice and the embryo investigators make their own judgments after consulting other experts in the field and reading extensively in the literature, they can learn well under this system and the companies can obtain valid data. The opposite may occur if the natural desires of company representatives to see their products succeed should influence the investigators or, worse still, if the companies should take on the job of writing the investigators' papers for them. It has been done; Senator Humphrey's committee turned up a case in which a physician asked the sponsoring company to write the report because he wanted to "be sure that the manuscript would come as close" to what the company wanted as possible![17]

When a new drug is first given to humans, the purpose is to detect gross toxicity and to see how its effects compare with those observed in the test tube and in animals. If these preliminary studies yield satisfactory results, further investigation included under Phases 2 and 3 involves the use of controls.

Whenever an investigator is studying a drug in humans he is consciously or unconsciously using a control. He is comparing the action of the drug with the action of some other drug or no drug at all under similar conditions. The comparison may be with patients he has treated previously, with another group of patients who are treated differently, or with a control group of patients deliberately set up for that particular experiment, matched in every way that he can match them so that they are identical with the patients who receive the drug except that they receive a placebo. (The word "placebo," which literally translated from the Latin means "I will please," originally meant a substance that was given to a patient for its psychological rather than its pharmacologic effect. In recent years it has also come to mean a substance given in a controlled experiment for comparison with a drug being tested. In such cases the placebo is fashioned to look as much like the drug as possible.)

Sometimes the patient is used as his own control; the drug to be tested is administered for a time, and another drug or a placebo is administered for an equal period. Even this must be done so that some patients get the drug first and some the placebo first. It is important that neither the doctor nor the subject know whether a potent drug or a placebo is being given, since a chance remark from a doctor or even the expression on his face may suggest to the patient the nature of the medication. This is called the double-blind method. Identical observations, whether clinical or laboratory, are made during both periods and the data evaluated at the end after the code has been broken.

Occasionally controls are not needed because it is possible to compare the effects of a new drug with what has happened in the past. Patients with endocarditis or tuberculous meningitis almost invariably died before the advent of the antibiotics. When recoveries occurred after treatment with penicillin and streptomycin respectively, doctors could be certain that these drugs were effective. In most studies of disease, however, controls are advisable, and in some they are imperative.

Yet even antecedent planning and employment of large numbers of subjects as controls do not assure that the matching will be correct. In a study of the effectiveness of pertussis (whooping cough) vaccine in school children conducted in Grand Rapids from 1939 to 1944, 4,789 children were vaccinated and 5,011 were followed as controls. But all this work went for nothing, because the vaccinated children were those whose parents asked for vaccination while the purported controls were children of the same age, sex, and area of residence who had not presented themselves for vaccination. One can assume that parents who brought their children for vaccination would likely be more zealous to guard their children's health in other ways, but more concrete discrepancies between the two groups were found. The control children had less exposure to pertussis in their homes, owing in part to the fact that 47 per cent of them were only children, as compared with 20 per cent among the vaccinated group.[18] Since it has been shown that pertussis is much more likely to be transmitted by exposure in the home than by outside exposure, the entire study was rendered invalid by this simple fact. The approved method today is the random selection of experimental subjects and controls.

Whether the patient is used as his own control or different persons are used as control and test subjects, the placebo is becoming an indispensable tool for many clinical tests. The long list of symptoms that patients report after receiving placebos, from headaches and lassitude to nausea, diarrhea, and even skin rashes, attests to the prevalence of psychological reactions attendant upon taking medication or merely focusing of attention upon health and illness. Also, placebos alleviate pain. Various studies have shown that from 21 to 39 per cent of patients were relieved of postoperative pain after taking placebos. They also relieve the pain of angina pectoris, the frequency of cough, and the symptoms of seasickness and anxiety.[19]

In addition to effectiveness as a check on the emotional reactions of the patient, the use of placebos also corrects for variations in the environment. If patients are randomly selected, let us say for a trial of measles vaccine, the same number of patients of each sex and of various ages and socio-economic backgrounds should fall in both the placebo and the drug-treated groups. Since cases may be more severe toward the end of an epidemic, a random method of selecting patients is needed to make sure that equal numbers of patients are treated with a placebo and with the drug during each part of the epidemic.

Controls are not always used when they should be. An analysis of a hundred articles in five leading American medical journals showed that controls had been employed in half of the studies, and only 27 per cent of them had been well controlled.[20] Although this analysis was done in 1951, the situation is far from perfect today. In a recent debate on the use of long-acting nitrates in the therapy of angina pectoris, it was pointed out that among more than three hundred articles on the subject in the medical literature, only eight were reports of double-blind studies; and among these, the ones that were carefully controlled demonstrated no advantage of nitrates over placebo therapy.[21]

Thus, in spite of the availability of complex and sophisticated methods, everything is not for the best in this best of all worlds of modern drug evaluation. For every good study there are dozens of defective ones. Directors of clinical investigation in pharmaceutical companies complain that investigators resent the suggestion that rigid control procedures be incorporated into the investigations; clinicians who pride themselves on the care with which they approach a diagnosis are often willing to use slipshod methods in trying out a new form of therapy, and most studies of drugs on ambulatory patients leave much to be desired. As Dr. René Dubos has said: "There are always men starved for hope or greedy for sensation who will testify to the healing power of a spectacular surgical feat or of a new miracle drug. They provide the testimonies of the new religions for which scientists with theories unproved or incomplete are always ready to provide the mystic language."[22]

Every group that tries seriously and objectively to assess the efficacy and toxicity of drugs on the basis of the information available is dismayed by the scarcity of carefully planned, adequately controlled studies. In a spot check of eleven new drugs on which comments of referees were requested by the Council on Drugs of the AMA (American Medical Association), I found that from four to eight consultants had made a report on each drug after reading the data on the clinical tests submitted by the nine drug companies sponsoring these drugs. The design and conduct of the clinical trials were commented on by fifty-one of the fifty-eight consultants. Only nineteen (or one third) of the comments were favorable, two were mildly critical, and thirty (or 52 per cent) were highly critical. The acting secretary of the same council reported: "Of the twenty-six new monographs added to the 1963 edition of *NND*, [*New and Nonofficial Drugs*, an AMA publication that will be discussed further in Chapter 9] it was deemed necessary in all but four instances to include some statement to the effect that the Council considered the available data to be inadequate or insufficient in one way or another."[23]

Data sent to the FDA provoke the same reaction. Dr. John O. Nestor of that agency testified: "Many new drug applications have been deficient in data necessary to establish the safety and efficacy of the drug. Often the evidence submitted is in the form of anecdotal or testimonial letters and, where individual case histories are furnished, they are lacking in necessary laboratory and clinical details. Far too few of the studies are adequately controlled."[24]

Considering the abundant opportunities and the profit in money or in notoriety, it is surprising that so few doctors succumb to the temptation of falsifying the data submitted to the drug company for transmission to the FDA. Nevertheless, one physician was recently reprimanded and fined after he had pleaded *nolo contendere* to the charge of submitting "false, fraudulent, and fictitious" reports on drugs.[25]

Certain entire fields of clinical testing have hardly been scratched. One of these is the efficacy and toxicity of drugs in children. Bitter experience in recent years has brought home to doctors that children react differently from adults to some drugs. The chairman of the Committee on Drug Dosage of the American Academy of Pediatrics went so far as to claim: "Usually we find the drug is unsuccessful for the small infant, the premature, when he becomes a dead monument to the drug."[26] In recent years such tragedies have shocked the medical profession into realizing that the infant can be injured by doses of drugs such as chloramphenicol and of vitamin K, which, given to adults in the same ratio according to body weight, would do no harm.

The hiatus between knowledge and need is even wider when we look at the production of congenital deformities by drugs. The thalidomide episode (see p. 200) opened a Pandora's box of problems and puzzles; yet we know so little about how and when such deformities occur, what chemical configurations cause them, and how congenital defects in animals relate to those that occur in man that we are still in a state of stunned bewilderment at the enormity of the problem.

Thus we see that all drugs should be thoroughly tested first in adults in whom there is no possibility of pregnancy. If there is good reason to use the drug in infants, young children, or pregnant women, careful clinical trials can then be initiated in these groups.

The design of experiments, the selection of patients and controls, and the interpretation of the results all should be carried out today in accordance with the accepted principles of statistics. Richard H. Shryock, the medical historian, has said that Pierre Louis's article published in 1835 was in some respects "the most significant study ever made in medical method."[27] Yet all Louis did was to list the patients with pneumonia treated by bleeding in a single Paris hospital, and those who had not been bled; then he compared the number of deaths in the two groups. There was no difference. Elementary? Yes, but it had not been done before!

Today we have progressed well beyond this point, and experiments with drugs are designed in such a way as to show that the result obtained is the effect of the drug under study and that the probability of its occurrence by chance is negligible. Readers of medical journals are conditioned to expect that pertinent statistical methods will be used. At least this is what the better-trained investigators provide and the well-informed readers expect, but we are still falling far short of the ideal. We would not agree with the Philadelphians who fined William Cobbett for slander when he used statistics to disprove Benjamin Rush's claim of curing yellow fever by bloodletting in 1793.[28] Yet, although we speak highly of statistics, our actions often belie our words. A recent analysis of the articles published in ten frequently read medical journals showed that in 25 per cent of the 292 articles evaluated no statistical tests had been applied, although they were necessary to support the conclusions.[29]

One word of caution is needed: statistics alone are not enough. They are ". . . merely a device for establishing the betting odds on the reproducibility of the results by mere chance. Statistical prognostication is always based on the assumption that the data used were worthy of collection; statistical analysis of poor data is tantamount to attempting to make a silk purse out of a sow's ear."[30]

Finally, after testing is finished and the data analyzed, the result must be reported to the medical profession. Comforting as this is to the author's ego and valuable as it can be to his reputation, these are not the main reasons for the report. Such communications are necessary so that doctors may use new knowledge in the treatment and prevention of disease and so that investigators may build still newer knowledge upon them.

The responsibility lies also upon editors of medical journals to reject or return for revision manuscripts that err in the treatment of data or the conclusions drawn. The editor pleads that he takes the best articles available but that he must fill up his pages. And so he must if every journal now being published is to survive. But should they? In recent years several medical journals have been started for no purpose other than as a vehicle for advertising—not that doctors aren't already deluged with advertisements, but somebody thought he could make money by flooding them with more. Since the volume of advertisements sold depends upon the number of readers, and readers depend upon a tasty bill of fare of articles, editors under these circumstances not only accept inferior articles, but often ask investigators to write articles that duplicate those written for another journal. I cannot see any advantage in so many medical journals, which crowd the shelves of libraries and stack up on the doctor's desk, surrounding the busy doctor with piles of printed matter and frustrating the conscientious doctor because he fears he may miss something if he doesn't read them all.

Make money, money by fair means, if you can;
if not, by any means money.
                        —HORACE, *Epistles*

There are no villians in the piece. . . . It is what
normal men and women find that they must and
will do in spite of their intentions, that really
concern us.
                        —GEORGE BERNARD SHAW,
                         Preface to *Saint Joan*

5

Economics of
the Drug Industry

The American drug industry has been the target of much criticism and some abuse in recent years. It has been called a money-grabbing monopoly that robs the purses of the sick and the aged to line the pockets of wealthy stockholders and highly paid executives. Drugs are said to be a big pill to swallow because of "prices which by any test and under any standard are excessive."[1] Critics claim that although much is spent for research in the drug industry, it produces mostly minor modifications of existing drugs and relatively few really new drugs. Competition in research is said to be misdirected, and competition by lowering prices nonexistent, whereas the "only real competition . . . is for the eye and ear of the physician—how many pages of advertising we can put out, how many samples we can distribute, how many detail men we can put in the field."[2] (Detail men are representatives of drug companies who call on doctors to persuade them to prescribe drugs sold by their companies.)

On the other hand, defenders of the drug companies point to the large number of new drugs introduced each year and to the speedy obsolescence of older drugs as they are displaced by new ones. They cite the rapid pace of the industry as a reason why the high profits from today's successes must be plowed back into brains and equipment. They contend that only by setting prices sufficiently above costs can capital be obtained for innovation, and that innovation is their practice and their salvation. They insist that not only is competition present, but that it is strenuous and unrelenting. Finally, they claim that they have an unparalleled record of public service—from educating doctors to flying life-giving serums to remote areas and donating tons of drugs to underprivileged countries.

Where in this welter of accusations and counteraccusations does the truth lie? How much is the drug industry contributing to society? Is it doing as much for the public as it should? As we have seen, most of today's drugs are produced by large corporations, not in the back room of the drugstore as they were a century ago. The firms that make drugs can be classified in several ways: according to the way they sell drugs—whether through doctors' prescriptions or directly to the public; by the kinds of drugs they make; or by their size and affiliations.

Companies that make drugs to be sold on the prescription of physicians and dentists are called prescription, or ethical, companies. Those who market drugs for sale directly to the public, or "over the counter," are called proprietary companies. But some ethical companies own proprietary companies and vice versa; and some large corporations own both kinds. For instance, Richardson-Merrell Inc. owns one proprietary firm, the Vick Chemical Co., and four prescription companies, among which is one of the oldest in the country, the Wm. S. Merrell Co. American Home Products Corp. includes three prescription companies and one proprietary company.[3] The Bristol-Myers Company, founded in 1887, concentrated on proprietary drugs, such as Sal Hepatica, very popular when this country was going through a wave of catharsis, and Bufferin, which is now riding high on the current wave of aspirin-gulping. In 1943 it bought the Cheplin Biological Laboratories, which under the name Bristol Laboratories moved into the prescription drug field, especially the production of penicillin products.[4]

The prescription drug industry is larger than the proprietary. Sales of ethical drugs for humans were valued in 1967 at over 2.9 billion dollars compared with 1 billion for proprietary drugs.[5] Also, the prescription drug industry is growing more rapidly; between 1947 and 1964 sales increased 311 per cent for prescription drugs and 162 per cent for proprietary drugs.[6] The more rapid growth stems in part from the more stringent regulation of the safety of drugs, which started around the beginning of this century and which drove off the market numbers of dangerous proprietary drugs. Finally, almost all drugs are first brought out as prescription drugs, and practically all of the research in the drug industry is done by a few prescription drug companies. They are the leaders; the others are the followers. Accordingly, in the sections that follow, we will be concerned only with the prescription drug industry.

The U.S. Bureau of the Census classifies companies according to whether they produce biological products, medicinal chemicals and botanical products, or pharmaceutical preparations. The first processes serums and other blood derivatives and vaccines. The second manufactures bulk chemicals or antibiotics or processes bulk botanical drugs. The third group puts the bulk chemicals, antibiotics, or botanicals into pharmaceutical preparations such as capsules, tablets, intravenous solutions, etc. in the proper form for consumption. The value of shipments of biological products in 1963 was nearly 96 million dollars; of medicinals and botanicals, nearly 306 million; and of pharmaceutical preparations, over 3.3 billion dollars.[7]

Again there is overlapping. Many small companies buy bulk chemicals and make appropriate preparations. Some make drugs in only one class, others in two or all three classes; Merck & Co., Inc., for instance, made bulk chemicals for many years, selling most in bulk and putting a few into pharmaceutical preparations. By a marriage of convenience with Sharp & Dohme it acquired a firm that had specialized in biologicals and had a large retail sales force. The American Cyanamid Co. arranged a propitious marriage of its Fine Chemicals Division, a large manufacturer of synthetic chemicals, with the Lederle Laboratories, which had long produced biologicals and vitamins. On the other hand, certain "old-line" companies, such as Parke, Davis & Co., developed biological and chemical production concomitantly. Other firms with good reputations stick to one area; G. D. Searle & Co. confines its activities to chemical drugs, and S. B. Penick & Co. deals only in botanicals.

Drug companies can also be classified according to size. The 136 firms that are members of the Pharmaceutical Manufacturers Association are the largest and make most of the pharmaceutical preparations in the United States. Table 2 is derived from a list of the sales, earnings, and assets of American drug companies that make detailed figures public. Only those firms are included that are members of the Pharmaceutical Manufacturers Association or are parent firms of members.

Among the companies dealing only in prescription drugs, the

TABLE 2. Sales, Earnings, and Assets of Leading Pharmaceutical Companies in 1967

Companies Marketing	Sales* Amount	Rank	Earnings* (after taxes) Amount	Rank	Total Assets* Amount	Rank
PRESCRIPTION DRUGS						
Eli Lilly & Co.	408,352	1	53,708	1	372,523	1
Abbott Laboratories	303,341	2	28,081	4	288,909	3
Upjohn Company	272,970	3	30,057	3	277,814	4
Smith Kline & French Laboratories	259,966	4	42,103	2	200,553	5
Parke, Davis & Co.	239,246	5	20,960	6	334,170	2
DIVERSIFIED DRUG PRODUCTS *(including toiletries)*						
American Home Products Corp.	987,252	1	104,072	1	601,640	1
Bristol-Myers Company	730,147	2	52,019	2	445,798	3
Warner-Lambert Pharmaceutical Co.	656,822	3	51,552	3	485,950	2
Squibb Beech-Nut, Inc.	577,945	4	40,076	6	437,947	4
Johnson & Johnson	525,771	5	41,163	5	371,880	5
CHEMICALS						
Union Carbide Corp.	2,546,000	1	170,686	1	3,088,339	1
Dow Chemical Co.	1,383,000	2	130,853	2	1,910,621	2
American Cyanamid Co.	937,000	3	70,308	4	910,440	3
Chas. Pfizer & Co., Inc.	637,776	4	58,255	5	657,936	4
Merck & Co., Inc.	528,126	5	89,314	3	456,390	5

* Figures rounded to thousands
SOURCE: *Drug Trade News*, September 23, 1968, pp. 11–12.

names of the top five, in order of sales (shown in the first section of the table), are practically household words in the United States.

Among those in the second section, which lists companies marketing diversified products, American Home Products Corp. owns three ethical drug companies: Ayerst, Ives, and Wyeth. Bristol-Myers owns the Bristol Laboratories, as has been mentioned. The Warner-Lambert Pharmaceutical Co. has two subsidiaries, the Texas Pharmacal Co. and the Warner-Chilcott Laboratories. Squibb Beech-Nut owns E. R. Squibb & Sons. Companies in this group may also have subsidiaries that make cosmetics, process foods, or manufacture other items far removed from drugs.

But it is among the third group, the chemical corporations, that the greatest diversification occurs; these companies are often industrial giants with large holdings in heavy and fine chemicals, fertilizers, and other industrial products. Among these many products, pharmaceuticals may play a small or a large part. Examples of the latter are the Lederle Laboratories, a major holding of the American Cyanamid Co. and Merck Sharp & Dohme, an important part of Merck & Co., Inc.

The American drug industry started as a number of small firms, often owned by a single individual who was usually a physician or a pharmacist. At first these firms merely sold the end products of someone else's manufacturing or made crude extracts of local herbs and minerals. As they gained technical skill, gathered trained personnel, and above all amassed capital, they began to improve the drugs and the methods of making them. Further growth brought with it the ability to do research, to make significant modifications of old drugs, and to search for new drugs. This pathway is still open today. Every once in a while a company that has been marketing individual or combinations of drugs that are already on the market will develop a research program of its own and head for the big time. A recent example is the A. H. Robins Co., Inc. In the words of its president: "We couldn't spend the money for research until we had it . . . and it wasn't until 1942—when our sales volume first hit the hundred thousand dollar mark—that we could think of changing our organization from a completely sales-minded operation to one which combined both research and sales." Their research group moved from rented quarters into their own building in 1952, and in 1957 they marketed methocarbamol, a muscle relaxant, the first product to be developed completely within their own walls.[8]

But this typical American success story does not apply to all. Obstacles, sometimes insurmountable, stand in the way of the small company's growth. Mr. Seymour N. Blackman said that his company, Premo Pharmaceutical Laboratories, Inc., was forced to sell its patent rights to drugs rather than market them itself, because it could not compete with the avalanche of advertising that the large companies can set in motion.[9]

Meanwhile, as the profits in the pharmaceutical industry burgeoned and the prospects of more success brightened, other corporations—manufacturers of chemicals or cosmetics, for instance—reached in to share the pie. As a result, many firms involved in the production of prescription drugs are large multi-million-dollar corporations arising either from original drug companies or more often by purchase or merger from the outside. The number of combinations in the drug industry rose progressively from sixteen in 1946 to seventy-four in 1965. During this same period, mergers with firms outside the United States rose to a peak of twenty-two in 1964.[10]

In the 1968 *Fortune* magazine list of the five hundred largest industrial corporations,[11] Union Carbide ranked 25th; Ling-Temco-Vought 38th; Dow Chemical 53rd; Colgate-Palmolive 81st; American Home Products 86th; and American Cyanamid 94th. Union Carbide, with assets of 3 billion dollars, owned one small prescription company, the Neisler Laboratories, which it subsequently sold for about 11 million dollars.[12] Ling-Temco-Vought and the Dow Chemical Co., billion-dollar corporations, each had one relatively small division that manufactured pharmaceuticals. In contrast, the three divisions of American Cyanamid that manufacture medical products, Lederle Laboratories, Davis and Geck, and the Fine Chemicals Department, play a large part in the over-all operation of the parent company. It is not until we come to Eli Lilly & Company, which was 209th on the list, that we encounter the first company manufacturing only prescription drugs.

Since the size of the leading companies continues to increase and each year sees new mergers and acquisitions, the relationship of the top management of large companies to the prescription portion of their business may be remote. The chief executives of the subsidiaries that make prescription drugs contend that their companies operate independently, except that their earnings go to the parent corporation. Yet if a higher set of ethics should be expected of a pharmaceutical company because it deals in a commodity so vital to health, it is difficult to see how this can be achieved under the system of remote ownership. When a vital decision has to be made involving an ethical code on the one side and profits on the other, the top executives of the parent firm cannot have the same understanding of and sympathy for the ethical code as executives exclusively associated with ethical drugs, who maintain close contacts with the medical profession and the research scientists.

To illustrate further the gap between top management and the medical and scientific professionals involved in the discovery and use of drugs, among thirty-one presidents, board chairmen, or comparable executives of member-companies of the Pharmaceutical Manufacturers Association for whom university degrees could be ascertained, sixteen had no degrees other than an A.B. or B.S., one had an M.S., one an M.B.A., and seven were lawyers. There were only one pharmacist, one Ph.D., and four M.D.'s in the group.[13] This is surprising in an industry that is strongly dependent upon research and considers itself auxiliary to the practice of medicine.

Because twentieth century industry is based upon the application of scientific knowledge, the origin of each important step forward is the laboratory. This means that scientists and technologists are key people. But it seems that the larger the firm, the more likely are the chieftains to be elevated through business or administrative rather than scientific channels. And the administrator has difficulty understanding the scientist. The creative urge, the instinct of workmanship, the desire to keep standards high, frequently clash with the object of smooth co-ordination of resources, of economical operation, and the need to "play it safe." Also, in a large company more echelons are likely to be interposed between the working scientist and those who make the important decisions. This is not, of course, a problem of industry alone; it is felt acutely in government and in universities, but in each instance size exacerbates it.

Finally, Dr. William Comanor, a professor of economics at Harvard University, has assembled evidence to show that research laboratories in moderate-sized drug firms produce more new drugs in proportion to their investments than either the very small or very large firms. He estimated the optimal size of a research group to be fifty to seventy-five professional workers.[14]

Another frequent corollary of bigness is the concentration of market power within an industry, although the ability of one or a few firms to dominate a market depends in large part on their size relative to the market rather than on size *per se*. Industrial concentration is usually measured in terms of the proportion of the assets, employment, or output of an industry accounted for by the top few firms. Economists consider concentration important because the degree of concentration generally affects the performance of firms in the industry. It affects the allocation of resources among firms and industries, the internal administrative and engineering efficiency of firms, the rate of innovation and technological progress, the level and stability of employment in an industry, and the distribution of income and of political and social power. Although concentration is an important determinant of market power, other important elements of the structure of an industry include barriers to entry into the industry, advertising and product differentiation, the nature of the buyers, and the growth in demand for the industry's product.

Two polar types of market organization are discussed in economic theory: *competition*, where there are many firms selling an identical product, where firms and resources can move readily in or out of the market, and where consumers, firms, and owners of resources are fully informed about prices and other conditions in the market; and *monopoly*, where there is only one firm in a well-defined market. In the first case, firms have no market power; they simply adjust their output in response to the changes in the costs of production and the conditions of demand and supply in the market. In other words, the performance of firms in a competitive industry is dictated by the market. Monopolies, on the other hand, are free to set their own prices and output and to make other decisions solely in their own interests. Frequently they are able to earn "monopoly profits." Such firms have the latitude or discretion to pursue whatever goals they wish, and the goals they select may conflict with what is best for society. No industries meet all of the theoretical requirements for pure competition or monopoly; they fall somewhere in between. But the more closely an industry approaches either of the polar types, the more likely it is to exhibit the kinds of performance described above.

Two intermediate types of market organization are usually identified: *monopolistic competition*, where there are many small firms selling differentiated but similar products (for instance, retail clothing stores); and *oligopoly*, where there are a few large firms selling similar products (which may or may not be surrounded by a number of smaller firms). The key characteristic of oligopoly is that firms recognize their interdependence. Thus, a given firm is likely to act in concert with the other firms rather than respond independently to market forces. The automobile industry is an example of a tight oligopoly, where there are a few dominant firms. The drug industry is an example of a loose oligopoly, where power is distributed among a somewhat larger number of firms.

A concentrated market structure causes particular concern because, in the words of the Department of Justice: ". . . a concentrated market structure, where few firms account for a large share of sales, tends to discourage vigorous price competition . . . and to encourage other kinds of conduct, such as use of inefficient methods of production or excessive promotional expenditures, of an economically undesirable nature."[15]

On the other hand, size assures the capital for efficient operation and the development of new products. Also, when a parent company manufactures chemicals for other purposes, some drugs may be discoverd incidentally. For instance, among the compounds that the American Cyanamid Co. turned over to their Lederle Laboratories for screening was one originally intended for use as a rubber chemical. Lederle scientists found that it had some antituberculous activity and, after making some six hundred analogues, developed ethambutol, which is a very effective antituberculous drug.[16]

Although over 1,300 companies market drugs, most of these are small, because the 136 members of the Pharmaceutical Manufacturers Association sell about 95 per cent of the ethical drugs in this country. More important, the 30 largest companies have about three fourths of the market.[17] Do the few large companies at the top have a concentration of power?

Table 3 shows a number of industries in which the concentration, as determined by the proportion of the market supplied by the four or eight largest firms, runs from very low to very high. It will be seen that the drug industry is more concentrated than companies making ready-mixed concrete, dresses, or furniture, but not as concentrated as those manufacturing steel, automobiles, or cigarettes. By this index, drugs occupy a middle ground of concentration along with milk, canned foods, and meat.

In a survey of thirty-three firms that were members of the Pharmaceutical Manufacturers Association between 1951 and 1963 and that had sales of 30 million dollars or more in ethical drugs in the United States,[18] the first five companies accounted for 49.1 per cent of the shipments of drugs in 1951 and 37.7 per cent in 1960. The next twenty companies had 48.2 per cent of the market in 1951 and 53.2 per cent in 1960, while the remaining thirteen had 2.7 per cent and 9.1 per cent of the market in 1951 and 1960 respectively. In the different classes of therapeutic products (such as antibiotics or diuretics) there were frequent shifts of position among the companies; in 1960 none was leading in more than three of twenty classes of products, and only two were in that category. On the basis of

TABLE 3. Per Cent of Shipments of Goods Manufactured Accounted for by the Largest Companies in Selected Industries in 1963

Industry	Number of Companies	Total Value of Shipments (million dollars)	Per Cent of Shipments Accounted for by: 4 Largest Companies	8 Largest Companies
Ready-mixed concrete	3,999	2,293	4	7
Dresses	4,577	2,411	6	9
Wood furniture (not upholstered)	2,937	1,858	11	16
Bottled and canned soft drinks	3,569	2,211	12	17
Poultry-dressing plants	842	2,241	14	20
Fluid milk	4,030	7,026	23	30
Pharmaceutical preparations (Drugs)	944	3,314	22	38
Canned fruits and vegetables	1,135	2,743	24	34
Meat slaughtering plants	2,833	12,435	31	42
Petroleum refining	266	16,497	34	56
Flour mills	510	2,177	35	50
Blast furnaces and steel mills	162	16,611	50	69
Motor vehicles and parts	1,655	36,181	79	83
Cigarettes	7	2,655	80	100

SOURCE: U.S. Department of Commerce, Bureau of the Census. *Statistical Abstract of the United States.* 89th Ed. (Washington, D.C.: 1968).

this study Jesse W. Markham, professor of economics at Princeton University, a spokesman for the drug industry, pointed out that the market share of the top five firms in 1960 varied from 45 per cent to 78 per cent, with an average of 61.5 per cent, in the twenty groups of products studied.[19] He contended that the industry-wide level of concentration for the drug industry was slightly lower than the concentration in United States manufacturing generally. Among the top thirty-three firms, the share of the market of the first five had decreased as compared with the share of the other firms in the group. But when the entire industry was considered for the period from 1947 to 1958, the percentage of the market accounted for by the twenty largest firms increased from 64 to 73 per cent at the expense of the smaller firms.

These methods of comparison leave something to be desired, since competition among drugs is limited strictly to drugs in the same therapeutic category. The committee chaired by Senator Kefauver inquired into the concentration of production in several therapeutic fields.[20] It found that seven manufacturers shared in the production of the cortisone group of hormones; six produced antidiabetic drugs; six, the various tranquilizers; five, the vitamins; nine, the antibiotics; and three, the sulfa drugs. Furthermore, in the case of twenty-seven of the fifty-one products investigated, all of the U. S. output was produced by one of fifteen companies.

But we are still not making the proper comparisons. Since the doctor prescribes for diseases and not necessarily by drug categories, the degree of competition can be viewed only in terms of the drugs that are best for any particular disease. I have listed some of these in Table 4. Pneumococcic pneumonia and streptococcic sore throat are perhaps the most frequent infections amenable to specific therapy. Several antibiotics are highly successful in these diseases—the various kinds of penicillin, the tetracycline group, or erythromycin. Eight companies in the United States made one or more of these in 1960, so that some competition was present, provided that the physician was aware of the several alternatives when prescribing. If the patient had had one of the rickettsial diseases, or meningitis caused by the influenza bacillus, the choice would have been narrowed to four drugs; these were made by four companies. On the other hand, if a patient's pneumonia had been caused by a mycoplasma (a type formerly called viral pneumonia), the physician should have selected one of the tetracycline drugs, which were made by only three companies. (Erythromycin has since been shown to be effective in mycoplasma pneumonia. At the time of the hearings it was produced by two companies, neither of which made tetracyclines.) If the patient had typhoid fever, chloramphenicol should have been chosen above all other drugs. This was made by only one company until the patent expired

TABLE 4. Concentration of Production of Certain Drugs

Disease To Be Treated	Drugs Used	Number of Companies Producing
Pneumococcic pneumonia	Penicillin group	7
or	Chlortetracycline	1
Streptococcic sore throat	Oxytetracycline	1
	Tetracycline	3
	Erythromycin	2
		(8)*
Rickettsial diseases (Rocky	Chlortetracycline	1
Mountain spotted, typhus,	Oxytetracycline	1
scrub typhus, or Q fever)	Tetracycline	3
or	Chloramphenicol	1
Hemophilus influenzae meningitis		(4)*
Mycoplasma pneumonia	Chlortetracycline	1
	Oxytetracycline	1
	Tetracycline	3
		(3)*
Typhoid fever	Chloramphenicol	1
Rheumatoid arthritis	Cortisone group	7
Childhood type of diabetes	Insulin	3
Mild, late-onset diabetes	Tolbutamide	2
	Chlorpropamide	1
		(3)*

* Figures in parentheses show the number of companies producing any one of the drugs in the group at the time of the subcommittee hearings.
SOURCE: Adapted from Chart 8 in U.S. Senate, Committee on the Judiciary, Subcommittee on Antitrust and Monopoly, 87th Cong., 1st Sess.: *Study of Administered Prices in the Drug Industry* (1961), p. 67.

in 1967. (From recent evidence it appears that a newer drug, ampicillin, introduced in 1964, is equally effective. It is marketed by four companies in the United States.)

For a patient with rheumatoid arthritis of such severity that it would not respond to aspirin or other milder drugs, the cortisone group of drugs might have been the proper treatment. These were manufactured by seven different companies. Diabetes mellitus is different, however, because the childhood type, if sufficiently severe, will respond to nothing but insulin, made by only three companies. Diabetes beginning late in life, if it is not too severe, might be favorably affected by one of the oral antidiabetic agents, in which case they would be the drugs of choice because of the discomfort of insulin injections. At the time of the subcommittee hearings, two such drugs were on the market; and these were manufactured by three companies, none of which produced insulin.

I could list many examples, but I think these are sufficient to show that there is some truth in both viewpoints. In the case of many drugs, unlike breakfast cereals, television sets, shampoos, or automobiles, a single drug or group of drugs is best; there is no second best. In many cases they are manufactured by only a few firms. On the other hand, in a disease such as ulcer of the stomach, the physician will rely strongly on diet and rest and will prescribe, in addition, a mild alkali to neutralize excess stomach acid. These he can choose from among a large number of drugs, and, since many are common inorganic salts such as calcium carbonate or magnesium oxide (milk of magnesia) upon which there are no product patents, they are made by a number of companies.

Concentration of the sales of drugs varies considerably, depending upon whether a drug, or the process of making it, is patented. As was shown in the Kefauver committee hearings, small companies who may wish to market drugs have no access to certain ones because the larger companies that manufacture them are not willing to sell to them in bulk form. At the time of these hearings, tetracycline was produced by three companies and sold by those and two others. Since then, a number of small companies have been able to obtain a supply from abroad. Chloramphenicol, produced by Parke, Davis alone, was sold only by Parke, Davis during the life of the patent. Among the corticosteroids, four brand name products accounted for more than 75 per cent of the market, and sales by small companies for 11 per cent.[21]

Granted that there is some concentration of drug production and sales in some areas, is this necessarily bad? For an answer, we need to turn to other factors that relate to competition. Firms compete by making new or better products; by selling them more cheaply; by making them more efficiently or by reducing profit margins; or by selling them more cleverly and aggressively.

Let us look at the nature and extent of each type of competition in the drug industry and try to judge its desirable and undesirable effects. I shall consider product innovation and efficiency in this chapter and prices and marketing in the next two.

What manufacturers call "new products" occupy a spectrum from life-saving breakthroughs at one end to a change from round to triangular tablets or the addition of peppermint to the flavoring solution at the other end. For purposes of discussion I have classified these into true innovations, pseudo-innovations, and minor variations. First let me describe them and then determine how many of each the drug industry has produced.

True innovations can be further subdivided into epoch-making advances and improvements of existing drugs. There are few really new drugs; when such drugs are introduced, they make history. Among the antibiotics, penicillin, streptomycin, and chlortetracycline were important advances. Oxytetracycline was no advance over chlortetracycline—in some respects it wasn't as good—but it was marketed as Terramycin just the same. I would call products of this kind pseudo-innovations. Others have called them "me-too" drugs. On the other hand, tetracycline represented a definite advance over chlortetracycline (and oxytetracycline) because it produces fewer adverse reactions and would be classified as an improvement of an existing product. Of course, it is possible to advertise a pseudo-innovation so that it sounds as if the man who devised it will get the Nobel Prize next week, and this we shall consider later, but despite a few differences on borderline drugs a remarkable consensus is seen whenever experts in the particular field are asked their opinion as to whether a drug is a real improvement or not.

New products in the third class, minor variations, are an attempt to make the products more attractive in form or flavor or easier to take. Flavor and solubility are sometimes important, sometimes not. Although an adult rarely complains of the taste of a medicine, in pediatrics taste many mean the difference between the drug's being swallowed or spit on the floor.

The Committee on Cost of Prescribing of the British Ministry of Health summarized the pros and cons of attractive medicines as follows:

". . . there is much to be said for making medicines sufficiently pleasant to be acceptable to patients and especially so if these patients are children. There is, however, nothing to justify making medicines excessively attractive (and possibly a danger to small children). Often these very attractive medicines are far more expensive than the alternatives . . . which . . . are sufficiently pleasant for all normal requirements."[22]

Complete dissolution of the drug is imperative when the drug is to be given intravenously, but whether aspirin dissolves in a glass of water in ten seconds or three minutes is of no consequence, despite television commercials implying that it is. The other factors associated with the effectiveness of the aspirin—the amount of food in the stomach at the time, the acidity of the stomach contents, and the activity of the stomach—are much more important and vary tremendously in themselves.

Minimal standards of stability and solubility are laid down in the official compendia, the *USP* (*United States Pharmacopeia*) and the *NF* (*National Formulary*).* The manufacturer must come up to these or run the risk of having his product seized by the FDA as misbranded. Thus, beyond a certain point, the claim that his drug is superior to that produced by his competitor is merely a lingering trace of the boastful exaggeration of the spieler in the old medicine show. On the other hand, it is important that a predictable quantity of the drug reach the site in the body where it is expected to act. Tests to measure this will be considered in Chapter 11.

To complicate the picture, new products consist not only of single entities, but also of mixtures of drugs. Rarely is a mixture an epoch-making advance. Mixtures of an estrogenic hormone and a progestogen used for the prevention of conception can be classified as such because they imitate the rhythm

* The word "formulary" means a list, together with preparations and dosages, of (1) widely used drugs, (2) recommended drugs, or (3) drugs that alone are approved for use. In this book the second definition is meant. Where the third definition is meant, the term "closed formulary" will be used.

of the secretions of the adult female. The first of these preparations on the market was given the trade name Enovid.

More often, a mixture may be an improvement of an existing product. For instance, a serious adverse reaction of the sulfa drugs was precipitation in the urine leading to the formation of stones that block the ureters (the tubes leading from the kidneys to the bladder). Because the solubilities of sulfa drugs in a mixture are independent of each other, when three of them are combined, each in one third the usual dose, kidney stones practically never occur. This observation justified the marketing of a mixture of three sulfa drugs. Ephedrine and similar compounds are used to reduce the swelling of the nasal passages that occurs in the common cold and hay fever, but they also produce nervousness and sometimes palpitation of the heart. These effects are commonly neutralized by including a small dose of a sedative, such as a barbiturate, in the preparation.

Most mixtures represent minor modifications of existing preparations. A few of these are justified because of convenience. When two drugs are frequently prescribed to be taken at the same time, it may be more convenient for the patient and he may be less likely to forget to take a dose if he has fewer doses to take, in other words, if the drugs are combined in one preparation. Such combinations, on the other hand, presuppose that the ratio of the two drugs in the combination will always be the ratio needed. This is not true. More often it is necessary to increase the dose of one drug without increasing the dose of the other, and thus a fixed ratio means that the patient will get either an inadequate dose of one or an excess of the other.

Sometimes two drugs are given together because they have a similar effect and each is thought to reinforce the other. Thus, caffeine has been given with aspirin for many years because both may reduce headache. A more recent practice has been to include in one tablet one of the chlorothiazide diuretics (which lowers blood pressure) and a hypertensive agent, such as reserpine (which acts on the central nervous system). Here again we run into the problem of comparative dosages. In the case of aspirin and caffeine, the doses have been established by long usage, there are wide limits of tolerance, and both drugs are relatively free from adverse effects. In the case of antihypertensive agents, however, adverse effects are more frequent, and the dose that some patients can tolerate without ill effects is strictly limited. Since the dose of each drug must be individually determined, the proper ratio for the patient will rarely match the ratio in the marketed preparations.

In summary, while rational medicine has greatly diminished the need for mixtures, sales promotion tends to perpetuate their use.

How do the drugs produced today measure up in terms of the above classification? Table 5 shows the number of new products, including mixtures, marketed in this country in the past nine years. In 1959, the peak year, there were 315 new products, of which only 63 were new single chemicals, while 49 were duplicates of existing drugs and 203 were mixtures. An additional 104 products represented new dosage forms of drugs already on the market. The number of drugs in each of these categories has decreased in the intervening years, in part no doubt as a result of criticisms voiced in the hearings of congressional committees and in the press, and stricter regulation by the FDA. For the period from 1959 through 1962, the year of the Drug Amendments Act, the average number of drugs in each group was two to three times as many as the average number in the subsequent five years.

The last line in the table shows the drugs introduced each year that were distinctly different from any previous drugs. The judgment as to which drugs should be included in this list was made by the consultants of the *Medical Letter* from 1959 through 1964. Using the same criteria, I have selected the drugs for subsequent years. The drugs in this group are shown in Table 6. It is apparent that the number of truly new drugs is small in comparison to the total number introduced and has been remarkably constant throughout the entire period. Adverse publicity and the new regulations seem to have caused a decline in the introduction of analogues and duplicates of existing drugs. The reduction in new dosage forms has been even

TABLE 5. Number of New Drugs Marketed in the United States

Year	1959	1960	1961	1962	1963	1964	1965	1966	1967	1968
Total new products*	315	306	260	250	199	157	112	80	82	87
New single chemicals*	63	45	39	27	16	17	23	12	25	11
Duplicate single products*	49	62	32	43	34	29	18	15	25	26
Compounded products*	203	199	189	180	149	111	71	53	32	50
New dosage forms* (not included above)	104	98	106	84	52	41	22	26	14	21
New original chemical entities*	32	30	14	10	7	6	4	7	9	7
Important therapeutic advances†	4	3	3	1	3	3	2	3	4	4

SOURCES: * Paul de Haen: *New Products Parade* 1968 (New York: Paul de Haen; January 1969).
† Figures for 1959–1963 from "Important Advances in Drug Therapy, 1959–1964," *The Medical Letter* (New York: Drug and Therapeutic Information; 1965). Figures for 1964–1968 compiled by the author. (See Table 6.)

TABLE 6. Important New Drugs Introduced in the United States—1959–68

Year	Drug	Therapeutic Class	Companies Marketing
1959	Griseofulvin	Antibiotic	Schering, McNeil, Ayerst
	Phenformin	Antidiabetic	U.S. Vitamin
	Thiotepa	Antineoplastic	Lederle
	Imipramine	Antidepressant	Geigy
1960	Methicillin	Antibiotic	Bristol
	Guanethidine	Antihypertensive	CIBA
	Glucagon	Blood-sugar regulator	Lilly
	Spironolactone	Diuretic	Searle
1961	Cyclophosphamide	Antineoplastic	Mead Johnson
	Vinblastine	Antineoplastic	Lilly
	Live poliomyelitis vaccine	Vaccine	several
1962	Fluorouracil	Antineoplastic	Roche
1963	Methyldopa	Antihypertensive	Merck Sharp & Dohme
	Measles vaccines	Vaccines	several
	Penicillamine	Copper-binding agent	Merck Sharp & Dohme
1964[a]	Ampicillin	Antibiotic	Ayerst, Bristol
	Dactinomycin	Antineoplastic	Merck Sharp & Dohme
1964[b]	Cephalothin	Antibiotic	Lilly
1965	Lincomycin	Antibiotic	Upjohn
	Indomethacin	Analgesic and anti-inflammatory drug	Merck Sharp & Dohme
1966	Gentamicin	Antibiotic	Schering
	Allopurinol	Anti-gout drug	Burroughs Wellcome
	Furosemide	Diuretic	Hoechst
	Amantadine	Antiviral drug	Dupont
1967	Clofibrate	Drug used to reduce blood cholesterol	Ayerst
	Clomiphene	Antisterility drug	Merrell
	Ethacrynic acid	Diuretic	Merck Sharp & Dohme
	Ethambutol	Antituberculous drug	Lederle
	Pentazocine	Analgesic	Winthrop
1968	Propanolol	Anti-arrhythmia drug	Ayerst
	Azathioprine	Inhibitor of the immunologic response	Burroughs Wellcome
	Desferoxamine mesylate	Iron-binding agent	CIBA
	Anti-Rh antibody	Drug used to prevent formation by a mother of antibodies to an Rh-positive infant	Ortho

SOURCE: Information for 1959–1964[a] from "Important Advances in Drug Therapy, 1959-1964." *The Medical Letter* (New York: Drug and Therapeutic Information, 1965). Information for 1964[b]–1968 compiled by the author.

greater. But the output of real innovations has not been affected. In other words, good basic research has continued to pay off. In fact, its effects have been even more evident as the output of the imitative drugs has diminished.

Thus very few single drugs or mixtures are epoch-making advances; some are worthwhile improvements of existing products; and most are either pseudo-innovations or minor modifications of products already on the market. Unfortunately the drug companies are geared to methods of promotion borrowed from other industries, which claim that each new product is a significant improvement over any existing product. One of their main promotional tools is product differentiation, the distinguishing of substitute products from one another by advertising. For the most part, therefore, the drive to compete is channeled away from true innovation and into promotion, which pretends that new drugs are innovations when they are not. This has been admitted by Pierre Garai, one of the drug industry's most eloquent spokesmen:

"No manufacturer of drugs can afford to restrict his production to genuinely significant pharmaceutical innovations. . . . It should therefore surprise no one that we find slight modifications of existing products marketed by the bushel, a veritable blizzard of parity products slugging it out as each company strives to extend its share of the market, endless polypharmaceutical combinations *of dubious merit*, and a steady outpouring of new chemical entities *whose advantages to say the least, remain to be established*."[23] (Italics mine.)

Thus the advertising man dismisses true innovation as an unimportant method of competition.

To summarize the results of competition in the drug industry, although the emphasis on competition by innovation has produced some important drugs, yet the public is forced to pay for much research of limited value. As will be seen later, it also pays for unnecessary advertising and promotion.

Another way of competing is to lower prices by increasing the efficiency of production. Galbraith has said that under the system of oligopoly it is likely that "prices will be an umbrella which efficient and incompetent producers alike will tacitly agree to hold at a safe level over their heads and under which all will live comfortably, profitably and inefficiently."[24] So far as I can see, this has not happened in the drug industry. Technical know-how and the desire to maximize profits have combined to reward the efficient producers; these have thrived and displaced or submerged the inefficient ones. Or the inefficient companies have stopped manufacturing because they could buy more cheaply elsewhere, and have concentrated on selling.

A more controversial area of competition is price competition, which will be considered in the next chapter.

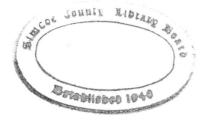

The drug industry story is a success story. But success cannot be accomplished through miracles. Unless the drug industry was given an opportunity to reap the harvests of its successes and to invest large portions of it in the development of its facilities and its research, this phenomenal success would not have been possible.

—SENATOR ALEXANDER WILEY

It is ironic that today only individuals imbued with an ideology of a crude "free enterprise" or with Marxism believe that the goals of a large corporation can be summed up simply in profit maximization.

—HAROLD L. JOHNSON

The real guarantee of nonstatist industrial organization in America is a substantially satisfied public.

—ADOLPH A. BERLE, JR.

6

Prices
of Drugs

In times of escalating prices, everything seems to cost too much, but since drugs are important to everyone's welfare and are often needed by those who can ill afford the barest necessities, a charge that drug prices are higher than they should be must be examined thoroughly. Are drug prices too high? No, says the drug industry. And they give as reasons for their answer: prices of drugs are actually low and are decreasing; the value in terms of health is great in proportion to the prices charged; drug companies take enormous risks and accordingly are entitled to high returns; and large profits are needed to finance new research adequately. For each of the reasons put forward, the critics of the drug industry have answers. Let us take up each of these points in turn.

First, in contending that drug prices are not really high, the drug industry points to the statement of Arthur M. Ross, commissioner of the Bureau of Labor Statistics, that the relative prices of the prescription drugs listed in the Consumer Price Index declined from 102.6 in 1960 to 89.6 in March 1967, as compared with an increase of 11.9 points in the index for all items during this period. Likewise, the Pharmaceutical Manufacturers Association Index of Wholesale Prices of Ethical Pharmaceuticals also declined from 100 in 1959 to 92.6 in 1966.[1]

In reply, the critics of the industry contend that prices have often been stuck at one level. For instance, Professor Henry Steele of the University of Houston showed that whereas the prices of penicillin and streptomycin (antibiotics that are available for production and sale to many firms) were lowered progressively until by 1960 they were sold for only 4 per cent and 11 per cent of their 1950 prices respectively, in contrast the prices of three other antibiotics, each of which was monopolized by a single company, followed a different pattern. During the same period, the prices of chlortetracycline and chloramphenicol dropped from $8.00 for sixteen capsules to $5.10 (or to 64 per cent of the original price), and that of oxytetracycline from $8.40 to $5.10 (or 61 per cent). Then, from November 1951 to 1960, the prices of all three of these competing products remained at $5.10. In this connection a district court, on December 29, 1967, convicted three firms of having conspired to fix prices of tetracycline drugs.[2]

The critics also point out that identical drugs are sold by American firms much more cheaply abroad than in the United States. Differences in the relative purchasing power of the pound sterling and in per capita income could not account for prices for drugs in Great Britain at less than 40 per cent of prices for the same drugs in the United States.[3] To refute the evidence of the Consumers Price Index, the critics contend that this index is based on very few drugs and includes factors other than the cost of the product that influence the price of the product, such as the overhead costs of retail drugstores. In contrast, the average price of prescriptions rose from 36 to 57 per cent between 1954 and 1965.[4]

What are we to make of these conflicting opinions? Simply this. Whether drug prices are actually increasing or decreasing is not the main question. Economists would ask a more important one: Are the prices reasonable? And they would judge reasonableness by the difference between prices and costs (i.e., the profit). Since it is often difficult to determine the costs of producing a single drug, the profits of a firm or of the entire industry are often used instead. In competitive industries prices tend to be driven down to levels that produce reasonable profits by the actions and interactions of the individual firms. If prices are too high (well above production costs) some firms will cut prices to get more business, and the others will be forced to follow. But this type of price competition is infrequent in oligopolistic markets. In the drug industry price competition is not the usual practice because monopolies are created by the ownership of patents and by the fixing of trade names in the minds of pre-scribing physicians, and because the high costs of promotion make it difficult for small firms to enter the market. Thus the factors that tend to force prices down have not been character-istic of the drug industry.

As a second point in rebuttal, the drug industry asks: What

should be the price of health? Are drugs too high when they save lives and shorten illnesses? One of its spokesmen made up a balance sheet with the pneumonia of today on one side along with "$15 to $30 for drugs and just two or three visits from the doctor," and, on the other side, yesterday's pneumonia and "five weeks of hospitalization, long convalescence, and several hundred dollars for doctors, nurses, oxygen, and hospital care."[5]

Aside from the fact that the choice of a disease was not apt, since the best drug for pneumonia, penicillin, was not discovered in an industrial laboratory, this argument can be answered by looking at the prices of other commodities. Milk, bread, and shoes are also necessities, but competition has kept the prices down so that the public gets more than its money's worth. One economist explained that the end result of charging the customer according to what a product means to him is "just the monopolistic practice of charging what the traffic will bear."[6] Such a practice cannot be tolerated when it means that high prices prevent some people from buying drugs they badly need.

A third reason given by the drug industry for maintaining prices above barely competitive levels is that profits should be high because the risks are high. According to Dr. Jesse W. Markham the particular risks of the drug industry are: (1) quality control problems, (2) unanticipated adverse effects, (3) the discovery that misuse causes social problems, and (4) product obsolescence.[7]

Since drugs, of all products, must be safe, the first three of these risks are particularly pertinent, but precisely for this reason drug companies maintain elaborate systems for quality control and test drugs thoroughly for adverse reactions and other untoward possibilities. Also, the strict regulations of the FDA for inspection of plants and testing of drugs are a protection to the drug firm. These internal and external precautions should reduce the risk to manageable proportions. If not, the regulations should be made more strict until the risks are on a par with other industries. This will protect the drug firm, but more importantly the patient, because rather than money he risks health and life if the drug he takes is not safe.

Actually, the costs of quality control are not great. Professor William S. Comanor found that among twenty-one large drug firms in Canada, many of whom were subsidiaries of United States firms, expenditures for quality control accounted for only 3.6 per cent of the total cost of producing a drug.[8]

Regarding Markham's fourth point, there is no question that drugs become obsolete rapidly. Many examples can be cited. Among the adrenal steroids, cortisone was replaced by hydrocortisone and that by prednisone, dexamethasone, triamcinolone, and others. Chlortetracycline was partially replaced by oxytetracycline and tetracycline, and these, in turn, by demecycline and other analogues. Yet optimal results can be obtained with prednisone among the adrenal steroids and with tetracycline in its group of antibiotics; the other analogues merely gild the lily. Much of this obsolescence is brought on by the short-sighted practices of marketing imitative products that represent no real difference from existing drugs, and of claiming by misleading advertising that they are different. If price competition were increased, if patents on drugs were granted solely for genuine therapeutic advances, and if doctors could distinguish between real improvements in therapy and advertising puffery, rapid obsolescence of drugs would be much less frequent. The remedies for excessively rapid obsolescence lie with the drug industry; yet the spokesmen for the industry have consistently opposed them.

Even if one accepts the risks of the drug industry as they exist today, however, the total risk does not appear to be great according to Dr. William F. Mueller, chief economist of the Federal Trade Commission, who stated: "Losses, or even low profits, are practically unheard of among large drug companies. In this respect the drug industry is unique among important American industries." Among twenty-nine top companies, earnings fell below 5 per cent on investments only 0.4 per cent of the time. He also quoted the practical experts in risk, the stock analysts, as classifying the drug industry as a rapid-growth, high-profit, and "depression-resistant" industry.[9] To a hardheaded investor, that wouldn't sound like much of a risk.

Finally, the drug industry stakes its case on the need for profits to spark new research. Certainly no one can deny that profit has this function; the question is: How big a profit? Unusually high profits may cause a company to coast, to depend upon the drugs it has already innovated rather than to push vigorously to find new ones. Some observers point out that Parke, Davis's seventeen-year monopoly on chloramphenicol coincided with a period in which it introduced little or nothing of importance to the drug market, in contrast to its past excellent record for research and in contrast to the productiveness of other firms of similar size during the same seventeen years.

More importantly, while reasonable profits are needed to attract capital, profits need not be above a certain level to achieve this purpose. In 1966 the profits of the drug industry topped those of nearly all other industries at 20.3 per cent of net worth. Dr. Leonard G. Schifrin, Director of the Department of Economics at William and Mary College, testified that such profits are unfair to the consumer: "To justify a high price because it is necessary for future research is in fact to charge the consumer twice for the research. He is paying for the present research and future research." And charging the consumer twice means that the consumer pays the stockholder twice, once in dividends and again in plant and equipment; these are added to the stockholder's holdings, although the investment comes out of the patient's pocket.[10]

Thus we are bound to conclude that the claims made to justify excessively high prices and high profits in the drug industry do not hold water when examined carefully. Let us look next at how these prices have been kept at high levels.

It is an elementary principle in economics that when people want more of a product, its price rises, provided the supply remains constant; and when the demand for a product decreases, the price goes down. Likewise, if the supply increases while the demands remains constant, the price drops, whereas the price rises if the supply diminishes. This is what happens in markets that are reasonably competitive.

We have seen that the drug industry is an example of imperfect competition; thus drug companies are partially freed from pricing drugs according to the forces of supply and demand. Instead, most of the prices of drugs are administered prices. These are prices that are set on other bases than cost alone and are maintained for some period of time in spite of changes in supply and demand. In testimony before the Kefauver Committee, Dean Eugene Rostow of Yale University, speaking as a witness for the pharmaceutical industry, defended the practice thus: "In the most competitive markets we know anything about, the prevailing price at any given moment of time should have no fixed or determinative relation whatever to cost."[11] The reasons why companies set prices administratively are, in the short run, to attain a specfic return from a particular investment or to attain a specific percentage of the market for a particular product. In the long run, adhering to administered prices lessens competition in the area of prices, since the companies having most of the market tend to set an identical price for the same or similar products; this shifts competition to other arenas, such as product differentiation and innovation. Finally, setting prices above actual costs builds capital for research and makes the inflow of these funds more consistent.

Price competition does occur in the case of drugs that have been on the market for so long that patents have expired and the impact of brand names is less. Phenobarbital is a good example. It was originally sold under the trade name of Luminal; when the patent expired, the originating company still sold it under this name at a price considerably higher than that charged by companies marketing it under the generic name. But gradually physicians became accustomed to the name phenobarbital, so that today in this country practically all of it is sold under that name. On the other hand, the majority of drugs, and especially the newer drugs, are prescribed by brand name, because these trademarked names are persistently dinned into the doctor's ears. Competition among the vendors of these drugs involves attracting the doctor's attention rather than sparing the patient's pocketbook.

Suggestions for lowering prices have included prescribing

drugs by generic names; abolition or curtailment of patents on drugs; and more knowledgeable and skillful purchasing practices.

Names of drugs include the chemical name; the proprietary, trade, or brand name; and the nonproprietary or generic name. A drug commonly used in mental disease has the chemical name 2-chloro-10-[3-(4-methyl-1-piperazinyl)propyl] phenothiazine. Because such a name, although exactly descriptive of the drug, is impossible to remember and pronounce, the drug company coins a simple name for which it obtains a trademark; in this case, Compazine. Since only the owner can use the trademark, another name is also adopted, which will describe this drug no matter who is making or selling it. This is called the generic name, or the nonproprietary, official, or established name. For the drug in question the generic name is prochlorperazine. The processes of naming drugs will be discussed in Chapter 9. For the present, let us look at the relation of names to price.

When a company discovers a drug or obtains from someone else the right to market one, it wants the doctor to use its product. To do this, it gives the drug a simple and catchy trade name; then, with all the sales techniques it can muster or is willing to pay for, it tries to inform, persuade, cajole, insidiously suggest, or loudly and incessantly bombard the 300,000 practicing doctors so that the name sticks in their minds whenever they have occasion to prescribe that drug. Of course, the company could elect to sell the drug under its generic name and compete mostly by price, but this is rarely done. Reserpine, which is commonly used in the treatment of high blood pressure, is an exception. It is sold to the druggist under the trade name of Serpasil by CIBA for $23.50 per thousand tablets; yet Vita-Fore Products Co., Inc., sells it under the generic name for $.70 per thousand.[12]

When there are many brand names for a drug and doctors are prescribing by brand name, the druggist must store them all and thus increase his investment and add to his overhead. It is no wonder that many people have insisted that prescribing by generic name is the solution to the problem of the cost of drugs to the patient.

The drug industry has arguments against this seemingly simple solution. It points out that the higher prices of drugs sold under trade names include the costs of research, which must be recouped so that research on other drugs may follow. It contends that the companies that sell by generic name only are doing no research and contributing little to the conquest of disease. While this is sometimes true, it does not explain, for instance, why Upjohn also sells reserpine under a trade name (Reserpoid) and charges $19.98 for a thousand tablets. Who did the research that produced the drug? Unfortunately for their argument, the drug companies are unable or unwilling to produce the evidence showing the costs of the research that led to the discovery of a particular drug. Perhaps it is impossible, but it does not help the unbiased observer make a judgment.

Another reason given for prescribing by brand names is that a single drug is formulated in different ways. These involve the size of the particles of the drug, the substances with which the drug is combined, and the coating of a tablet or capsule. Industry spokesmen point out that the official compendia that set the standards for drugs in the United States, the *USP* (*United States Pharmacopeia*) and the *NF* (*National Formulary*), were established at a time when drugs were put in final dosage form by the local pharmacist, so that these compendia "do not cover the complex processes of modern mass production, and they give relatively little guidance to standards in this area. Neither do they cover other considerations of great importance to modern production and distribution, such as long-term stability."[13] Furthermore, spokesmen for the larger drug firms claim that some drugs are prepared so poorly as to be insufficiently absorbed from the intestinal tract, and imply that brand names are an index of reliability.

In the jumble of claims and counter-claims, certain facts seem clear. With respect to quality control, the FDA tests every batch of an antibiotic or of insulin individually, so that there is no question of the quality of these drugs. Yet one hundred 200,000-

unit tablets of penicillin are sold by Squibb, under a brand name, for $6.62 and by Pennex Products Co. under the generic name, for 92 cents.[14] Also, some products marketed by large and reputable firms, as well as those marketed by smaller and less well-known firms, have been seized by the Food and Drug Administration because they were contaminated with other substances, were of low potency, were wrongly labeled, or for some other reason required removal from the market.[15]

Although changes in formulation of a drug may affect its absorption from the intestines and hence its effectiveness, this is not a problem with all drugs. Digitalis, the mainstay in the treatment of heart disease for two centuries, has been carefully standardized for animals and for people, so that proper formulations are available to all comers. (It is interesting in this connection to see that one company, Davies Rose Hoyt, which markets digitalis under a brand name, charges $18.40 for a thousand tablets, whereas Lederle and Merck Sharp & Dohme, two of the largest companies, market it under the generic name and sell the identical quantity and dosage-form for $2.50.)[16]

Another example where the speed of absorption is unimportant would be ferrous sulfate, a salt of iron used in anemias that follow blood loss. Since only 20 to 30 per cent of a dose of iron is absorbed from the intestines, variation among different preparations of ferrous sulfate would make no appreciable difference in the amount reaching the blood stream; actually, the limiting factor is the amount of drug the patient can tolerate. Although differences in efficacy are negligible, differences in price are not; a thousand 0.3 gram ferrous sulfate tablets sell for $9.00 wholesale if bought as Feosol (Smith Kline & French's brand name) and for $1.32 per thousand as American Quinine Co.'s generic preparation.[17]

For some drugs, differences in absorption are important; more information must be obtained on how these are absorbed. The Task Force on Prescription Drugs of the Department of Health, Education and Welfare recently concluded that "if the active ingredient in two or more chemically equivalent products reaches the blood (or other fluid or tissue)—and becomes biologically or physiologically available—at the same time and in the same amounts, their therapeutic effects will be essentially the same."[18] The FDA and other groups are investigating the differences in the absorption of different formulations of identical drugs. As discussed in Chapter 11, differences in absorption have been found among the different preparations of certain drugs. It is important, therefore, that studies on physiologic availability be pushed vigorously.

Prescribing by generic name is desirable not only because it will save money for the doctor's patients, but also because it will identify exactly the product his patient is to receive. In my experience the multiplicity of trade names for a single drug confuses the physician and sometimes causes him to make therapeutic mistakes. Also the trade name does not guarantee that his patient will get the same preparation in February that he got in January. A drug company can change the ingredients in a preparation and retain the same trade name. A good example is a commonly used noncaloric sweetener, Sucaryl. This originally consisted of salts of cyclamate; later it was modified by the producer so as to contain saccharin in addition to cyclamate, although still sold as Sucaryl.[19] Such changes cannot be made under a generic name unless the official standards have been changed.

Most drugs are still protected by trademark and are sold only under brand names. Seventy-two per cent of the 409 products used most widely by persons aged sixty-five and over were in this category in 1966.[20]

In summary, at present the physician can prescribe certain drugs by their generic names with the assurance that whatever brand his patient uses, the effects will be similar. For these drugs I urge that he prescribe by generic name. When sufficient information becomes available on the other drugs, the doctor will be in a position to prescribe all drugs by generic name, and should do so. This will make for less confusion in prescribing and, when more than one company markets a drug, will usually save the patient money.

Another proposal to reduce prices is the abolition of patents on drugs. The majority report of the Subcommittee on Antitrust and Monopoly of the United States Senate stated:

> *Of the 17 foreign countries for which usable price information was obtained for the subcommittee by the Department of State, 6 grant patents of pharmaceutical products while 11 do not. . . . Of the 6 foreign countries for which price information has been obtained and which do grant product patents, 4 (Australia, Canada, Great Britain, and India) have compulsory licensing provisions. Moreover, 2 of these countries (Australia and Great Britain) will not issue patents on any mixtures of known ingredients. Thus, of these countries, only Belgium, Panama, and the United States grant patents on drugs without imposing any of these limitations or safeguards to the public welfare.*[21]

Abolishing patents has been vigorously opposed by representatives of the drug industry, who claim that more drugs have been discovered in recent years in the United States than in any other country and that this has been the result in large part of our patent system.

No doubt this country has been a leader in discovering drugs in recent years, but surely we are dealing here with more than one variable. America has also had the greatest resources to finance the drug industry. It has had the largest supply of trained personnel, and if we are to believe the complaints of the "brain-drain" from Great Britain, America's higher salaries, higher standard of living, and superior facilities for research continue to attract foreign scientists to this country. Finally, America has the largest number of top-flight universities whose scientists are working in fundamental areas relating to drugs. Many of them have been teachers of drug company scientists, and many of them function as consultants to industry. Thus it is not possible to pinpoint any one factor, such as the patent system, and claim this as the reason for an alleged superiority in the discovery of drugs.

Furthermore, much of the research in the drug industry is directed toward minor modifications of existing drugs. Of course molecular manipulation is important and should be pursued, but when it becomes obvious that a modification is yielding something that is no better than an existing drug, energies should be channeled back toward modifications that would be substantially different. The present system of granting patents freely for modifications that do not represent real progress is not in the public interest because it gives profits to the noninnovator as well as to the innovator and because it draws funds and skilled personnel away from more worth-while research.

Nevertheless, the record of achievement in the discovery of drugs is sufficiently good that we do not want to tamper casually with the present system. One reasonable solution is compulsory licensing of a drug after it has been on the market for several years. Although representatives of the drug industry claim that such a requirement would diminish the incentive for producing new drugs, this is unlikely, since royalties could be priced so as to yield reasonable returns.

Furthermore, as Professor Comanor pointed out, even if research in industrial laboratories were decreased by a system of compulsory licensing, basic research would more likely be diminished than applied research. But, he argued, basic research is precisely the area in which government, university, and other private laboratories have an advantage over industrial laboratories, because basic research requires an atmosphere of freedom of inquiry, which is hard to achieve in an industrial organization. Also, since most of the basic research is now done in university and government laboratories, it would not be difficult for them to take over industry's fraction. I would add that fundamental research thrives best where younger and older scientists are working side by side—in other words, where there are students, as in universities and in the laboratories of the National Institutes of Health. At the same time, research in such a setting serves to increase the supply of sorely needed professional workers.[22] For all of the reasons given, it appears that the public good would be best served by requiring companies to license a drug, after a reasonable period of time, such as three years, to applicants who were willing to pay a suitable rate of return. Such a system would force drug companies to compete, after an initial period of protection, on the basis of price or to devise a better product—both optimal social goals.

Accordingly, I would urge immediate implementation of the recommendation of the Task Force on Prescription Drugs[23] for a joint study by the several federal agencies involved, looking toward a revision of the patent and trademark laws on prescription drugs. I believe that the proper revisions would lead to a healthier public, a healthier economy, and a healthier drug industry.

Every prescription must be funneled through the doctor. He must either give the drug himself, order it given, or prescribe it for the patient to take. Thus if costs can be reduced by changes in prescribing habits, it is up to the physician to do it. But the physician has not been able to stand up against the barrage of advertising. As a spokesman for the drug industry has said: "Effective promotion, heavy promotion, sustained promotion has carried the day. The physicians have been sold. So has the country. . . . The best defense the physician can muster against this kind of advertising is a healthy skepticism and a willingness, not always apparent in the past, to do his homework."[24]

Amen! But what can be done to help him? I will make several suggestions:

1. More accurate and less misleading advertising.
2. Simpler generic names so that the physician can remember them better.
3. Dissemination of more information on drugs from unbiased sources.
4. Dissemination of more information to the physician regarding the prices of drugs.
5. More sophisticated purchasing of drugs.

The first will be considered in the next chapter; the second in chapters 9 and 11 on the AMA and the FDA; and the third in Chapter 13. Let us therefore consider the last two suggestions.

Information on the prices of individual drugs is easily obtained by picking up the telephone and calling the neighborhood druggist. I have found him always accommodating in this and other matters. But such calls take time; they cannot be made every time a physician prescribes a drug.

Alternatively, the physician can consult a list of prices, such as the one in the *Handbook of Prescription Drugs* by Dr. Richard Burack,[25] and specify the cheapest brands from among those that he considers reliable. He can do this by writing "Digitalis— Lederle" or "Digitalis—Lilly" (or Merck or Parke, Davis) according to his choice. He should also encourage his patients to shop around to obtain the lowest price for the brand or generic preparations he has prescribed. Purchasing by hospitals or other groups can be even more effective in lowering prices and will be considered later.

The physician will find an ally in the neighborhood druggist. If together they decide that an inexpensive brand of a drug is acceptable, the druggist can stock it and the physician can prescribe it by the company's name. But there's the rub: most physicians and pharmacists are in no position to pass on the quality of the drugs. Likewise the lone patient, presenting his prescription to the corner druggist, is still a rather powerless purchaser. Some larger group is required to marshal the expertise needed to determine the quality of drugs and to bargain with the seller on more nearly equal terms. Examples of this in the United States are purchases by federal, state, and local governments and by large hospitals.

The federal government makes large purchases of drugs for the military services and the Veterans Administration hospitals. The Defense Supply Agency expended 55 million dollars for drugs in 1962, and the Veterans Administration 28 million dollars. Drugs are also purchased by other federal agencies. The Defense Supply Agency inspects the plants of manufacturers who wish to sell to it and obtains sealed bids from contractors so that drugs can be purchased from the lowest bidder, provided quality is satisfactory. In only 5 per cent of instances where information relating to the quality of drugs was requested did the manufacturers refuse to comply.[26] An Interagency Procurement Advisory Council on Drugs was formed in 1962 to obtain and exchange information with regard to the quality, effectiveness, and adverse effects of drugs and to compare purchasing methods.

State, county, city, and some private hospitals also have facilities for balancing the price and quality of drugs. They have physicians on their staffs with extensive experience in the use of drugs, and these experiences can be pooled for the benefit of all. The pharmacists in the hospitals are familiar with the physical and chemical attributes of drugs they have handled, have a knowledge of the companies that generally manufacture drugs of high quality, and are knowledgeable about prices. Often there are investigators in hospitals who have studied some of the drugs before they are marketed. Pooling of this information leads to better purchasing. Moreover, the purchaser of large quantities is in a position to bargain for the best price among the companies marketing the same or essentially similar drugs. Mass purchasing has resulted in lower prices of drugs in the past; as health care becomes progressively more organized, and as people recognize the benefits of mass purchasing, it will become a greater factor in lowering drug prices.

Aside from the physician, it is important for the public to be aware of the differences in drug prices. To be properly educated in this area, the man on the street should be aware that although quality is paramount, there are substantial differences in price among drugs of the same quality and effectiveness. His interest in price when he talks to his physician and to elected officials will be reflected in greater awareness of the importance of price on all sides.

Do these recommendations for reducing the price paid for drugs, where feasible, mean that the company that contributes in research leadership, in efficiency of production, in better distribution of drugs, or in the dissemination of truthful information about them should not be rewarded for its efforts? By no means. There has been a conflict in attitudes that was neatly summarized in an exchange between Senator Kefauver and the president of Merck & Co., Inc.

"Senator Kefauver. The public interest comes in some place.

"Mr. Connor. It is our property right that has emerged from a research program which we supported with our stockholders' money."[27]

Industry spokesmen believe that when a board of directors decides to back a research program by risking company funds, which are in essence stockholders' money, and when the venture is successful, they are entitled to distribute the gains to the stockholders or to risk them further in the hope of still more gains.

If the changes that I have suggested are made, competition will be redirected along lines that should bring greater benefits to the public. The incentive will be increased to produce more worthwhile drugs, not fewer. If profits continue at a reasonable rate, they can be distributed as dividends, which will make it possible to attract new venture capital when this is needed. Or they can be plowed back into more plant equipment and personnel, thus compensating the shareholder by adding to his capital investment. In the unlikely event that profits in the future will not be great enough to do either, the government can share the cost of research where the risk is high or the returns are likely to be low. Since so much remains to be done to improve the health of the American people, and since their good health is a national asset, it is only fitting that some of the venture capital should be furnished by the people at large. As has been pointed out in Chapter 2, the federal government is already doing this, especially in cancer research and the production of viral vaccines. A slight extension of the present investment by the government would take care of any deficit in research income in industry without upsetting the present balance between industry and government.

Indeed it might be argued that no institution had done more to circumvent the process and operation of rational thought in a free society.
—OTIS PEASE, in *The Responsibilities of American Advertising.*

. . . we consider that if the industry is to assume the function of informing doctors about medicines . . . firms must discharge this role with appropriate responsibility. In our opinion this necessarily means that the industry must deny itself the wide license which is traditionally allowed to the advertisers of other commodities.
—THE SAINSBURY REPORT

7

Promotion of Drugs

Advertising of drugs is suggestive, misleading, sometimes downright false. It is aimed at the emotions rather than reason. It confuses, contravenes, and corrupts the physician. It ignores the patient's interests; at times it even causes injury to his health. And besides, it costs too much. These are some of the many criticisms directed against the advertising of drugs. In reply the drug industry has defended its practices with vigor.

One of its most eloquent spokesmen, an advertising executive, asked rhetorically, "Why all this drum-beating?" and replied, "The answer is quite simple. One, the drug companies cannot compete effectively without it. Two, it works. . . . Effective promotion, heavy promotion, sustained promotion has carried the day. The physicians have been sold. So has the country."[1] What can a dispassionate student of the subject make out of all this? Let us examine first some facts on advertising by the drug industry, second the criticisms in detail, and third the answers given by the pharmaceutical industry. Finally, I shall make some suggestions for improvements.

In 1958 the twenty-two largest drug companies spent 580 million dollars for promotion of drugs.[2] This represented 24 per cent of the receipts from sales of drugs compared with 6 per cent spent for research and development, 32 per cent for production, 11 per cent for general and administrative expenses, and 13 per cent for taxes, leaving a net profit after taxes of 13 per cent. It was estimated that the entire drug industry spent about 750 million dollars for promotional purposes. This amounted to more than three thousand dollars per year for each doctor in the United States—an island of doctors in a sea of advertising (some beleaguered doctors would say "at sea"). In the year beginning May 1, 1962, one general practitioner received 3,636 advertisements and samples promoting 604 different drugs.[3]

A little over half of the promotional expenses were for advertisements in medical journals and advertisements and samples sent by direct mail, and about 330 million dollars for the salaries and expenses of detail men.[4] It has been estimated that each visit to a doctor by a detail man costs nine to ten dollars. Advertising of drugs is therefore a big business and presumably good business. Is it also good medicine for the American people?

A staunch defender of present methods of drug promotion confessed:

". . . approximately three-quarters of a billion dollars is spent every year by some sixty drug companies in order to reach, persuade, cajole, pamper, outwit, and *sell* one of America's smallest markets—the 180,000 physicians. . . . And it is not too much to say that perhaps no other group in the country is so insistently sought after, chased, wooed, pressured, and downright importuned as this small group of doctors who are *de facto* wholesalers of the drug business."[5]

This pressure has not been suffered by doctors without a strong reaction. For instance, one protested that some of the methods used were "undermining sound medical care as well as degrading the reputation of the pharmaceutical industry and lowering the prestige of the medical profession."[6]

A frequent criticism is that drug advertisements are often misleading. A series of advertisements for tetracyclines, combined with a variety of substances purported to increase the absorption of these antibiotics, is a good example. The resulting barrage of advertising in which each company contended that its tetracycline product was absorbed best became known as the "battle of the blood levels." The battle turned into a comedy (with tragic overtones) when one of the companies, looking for the real cause of the differences in blood concentrations, found that certain fillers used in the capsules inhibited the absorption of the antibiotic into the blood, and that none of the substances that had been added improved absorption over that of the pure drug.[7]

Mr. William Goodrich, the assistant general counsel of the Department of Health, Education and Welfare for Food and Drugs, told a congressional committee that a drug called Clarin, which is an anticoagulant, heparin, formulated so that it can be taken by dissolving under the tongue, was advertised on January

14, 1961, in *The Journal of the American Medical Association* as being "of demonstrated value" in "post-coronary management" because, it was claimed, this drug had prevented recurrent heart attacks in a sufficient number of cases; yet the 1961 edition of AMA's *New and Nonofficial Drugs* said of Clarin: "However, there is as yet no convincing objective evidence that heparin, given sublingually, either prevents or ameliorates any manifestation of cardiovascular disease." Mr. Goodrich added that the drug was being prescribed for these unproved conditions, the total sales exceeding $300,000 annually.[8]

In one study, medical students read advertisements and later scientific articles about the same drugs. At the end of the course 74 per cent of the class were of the opinion that the drug manufacturer had tried to exaggerate the value of the drug 80 per cent to 100 per cent of the time, and 70 per cent believed it had tried to minimize the undesirable effects of the drug 80 per cent to 100 per cent of the time.[9]

Nor are the complaints confined to the United States. The editor of a leading British medical journal, the *Lancet*, complained: "An increasing proportion of the advertisements appearing in journals or distributed through the post have been clever rather than factual: they smack of the advertising expert rather than of the manufacturer himself. . . . Everybody now knows that skillful advertising can defy probabilities and sell almost everything to the public; but many of us feel that, where a serious profession is being approached on a serious subject, straightforward information is more suitable than the kind of ingenious persuasion nowadays so fashionable."[10]

A doctor writing to the same journal said flatly that unwarranted claims are made for many drugs "including vitamins, vasodilators, antispasmodics, tranquilizers, muscle relaxants, and hypotensive agents" as well as drugs for anemias.[11]

Advertisers want to change behavior. They found long ago that they could do this better by appealing to the emotions than to reason. This "intensification of feeling and the degradation of significance," as Walter Lippmann put it, has been transferred to medical advertising, as witnessed by the lavish displays in brilliant color, sometimes featuring scantily clad young ladies who appear too healthy to need the drug they purport to advertise. But this may be defended as a legitimate way of attracting attention. More important is the implication that the doctor is not up to date unless he switches to the latest wonder drug, which will either cure every infection, or make the chronically ill feel like a bridegroom that goeth forth to his chamber, or bring all of the endocrine glands back into working order overnight, depending upon the drug advertised.

The large number of drugs marketed, the conflicting claims that each one is better than the others, the emphasis on brand names, the rapid introduction of new products that are always said to be better than the old ones, and the sheer bulk of advertisements in the mails and in the medical journals (*The Journal of the American Medical Association* contains about six thousand pages of advertising a year, an amount which is exceeded by only one other weekly periodical, the *Oil and Gas Journal*[12])—all combine to give the doctor a sense of frustration and confusion, which coincides with the maxim that a former medical director of a drug company testified he learned from detail men: "If you can't convince them, confuse them."[13]

Furthermore, some advertising methods are such that they could be characterized mildly as in poor taste or, more strongly, as perverting the ethics of the doctors: such methods as employing medical students as detail men, sponsoring cocktail parties and golf matches, and giving expensive presents to doctors. Granted that the line between attracting attention and seducing is a fine one, these extremes are not worthy of an industry and a profession whose actions are so closely bound up with the health, the safety, and the lives of the public.

Another practice has been vigorously denounced: publicizing a new drug to the laity before it is thoroughly tested and sufficiently known to the profession. If the patient has read a sensational account of the miraculous cures of a new antirheumatic drug, who can blame him if he presses his doctor to prescribe it the next time he gets a pain? And if the doctor does not go along, he loses the patient to a doctor who will. Such articles in the lay press are double-barreled: they hit the stock market also. The author was surprised to have a stockbroker tell him confidently several years ago that Merck stock was going to soar in a few days because that company had just discovered a new diuretic, Diuril. I was already familiar with the properties of chlorothiazide (Diuril), but my statement that under no circumstances would I buy stock in a drug company about whose drugs I had prior professional knowledge was only received with an uncomprehending stare.

It is easy to multiply examples and to become indignant over the excesses and faults of advertisements for drugs. But we should also listen to the drug companies' side of the story. The defenses of the drug industry are that drug advertising gives important information and renders service to doctors; that the doctor does not have to pay attention to advertisements if he doesn't want to; that false, misleading, or tasteless advertising is infrequent; and that advertising as it is carried on is good business. Let us take them up in that order.

Physicians are busy men; everyone from the patient waiting in the doctor's reception room to the labor leader advocating state medicine agrees on that. Since they must "read as they run," bright, attractive, attention-getting, succinct statements about new drugs and new information on old drugs should be helpful. Some drug advertisements do this. If a doctor is to busy to read or if he has a specific question about a drug, it would be valuable if someone could tell him in a few words about the new drugs and answer his questions; detail men can perform these functions. As will be shown in Chapter 12, many doctors depend upon advertisements and detail men to alert them to the appearance of a new drug on the market.

A number of drug companies have a long record of manufacturing reliable drugs, of keeping adequate supplies available, and of providing information about them. Physicians have come to depend upon them. It is important that they be able to identify these firms and remember them.

Several companies have published monographs; a few of these have been factual, objective, and therefore educational. Some firms have produced films that dramatically portray the characteristics of a disease or the techniques of an operation. Some have sponsored seminars, lectures, or closed-circuit television programs for doctors. Finally, drug advertisements support medical journals, many of which would otherwise have to fold.

Let us look at the claim that the doctor must be alerted promptly to new developments in medicine. Even the most caustic critics of drug advertising admit that the doctor has little time to read. The actions of the doctor in response to the various sources of information available to him will be considered in a later chapter, but it is sufficient to note here that very few truly new drugs are produced, and those that are produced are brought to his attention promptly. Penicillin was not patented, and thus there was little reason to advertise it vigorously. There is no evidence that doctors adopted it any more slowly than they adopted the tetracyclines and chloramphenicol, which were proprietary products and were vigorously advertised.

Furthermore, alerting the doctor to the existence of a new drug without giving him at the same time a true perspective of its place in the spectrum of drugs may be a disservice. The advertiser says, "If we can get the doctor to prescribe a new drug the first time, his experience will tell him whether to use it again." This is the fallacy of superficial comparisons. When one is comparing soaps, the consumer, after one trial, can decide whether he will buy that brand again, since his decision depends mostly on his taste in colors, shapes, and perfumes. But an evaluation of a drug depends upon dozens, sometimes hundreds, of variables that are not intrinsic in the drug or its dosage, such as the time of day the drug was taken, what foods and drinks were ingested and when, whether the patient was taking other drugs concomitantly, whether he exercised afterwards, the general state of his health, the condition of his liver, his kidneys, and the organs that were directly affected by that particular drug, and, in addition, such obvious variables as whether the patient took the drug as directed or whether he took it at all.

Given these variables, the only accurate way to decide on the efficacy of a drug is to treat enough patients under conditions that will control as many variables as possible and to determine whether statistically significant differences can be obtained between patients who have received the drug and those who have not. This takes weeks or months, even in the clinics where patients with particular diseases abound; it is usually impossible in the average physician's practice. Prescribing a second time because the drug seemed to work the first time is usually prescribing by suggestion and not by reason. Nevertheless, reminder advertising should not be condemned entirely. It has its place, provided it is not expected to displace broader and deeper education about the drug and provided that education is available from other sources.

Is drug promotion educational? Since education signifies developing the faculties and powers of a person by teaching or instruction, a small part may qualify, but most of it is best labeled as inculcation, which means impressing by repeated statement or admonition. True education demands that the learner look at all sides, weigh the consequences, and choose the best answer; most advertising, whether it be by direct mail, journal advertisement, detail men, or thirty-page brochure, is calculated to impress upon the doctor that he should prescribe a particular drug.

Some detail men are conscientious and helpful in digging up facts about their drugs for a doctor who needs them. But lacking training in human anatomy, physiology, and pathology, and sometimes even in chemistry or pharmacy, they are ill-equipped to educate or even advise doctors. Besides, how can they free themselves from bias? As a writer in *Fortune* (a magazine that could hardly be accused of being anti-industry) pointed out: ". . . most detail men are paid on a salary-plus-bonus basis—an arrangement that scarcely encourages them to knock their own merchandise."[14]

Perhaps it was this kind of incentive that allegedly impelled a representative of Parke, Davis & Co. to tell Dr. Albe M. Watkins that chloramphenicol, which several expert committees have agreed sometimes causes aplastic anemia,* was "a perfectly safe

* Aplastic anemia occurs when the bone marrow does not manufacture an adequate number of red cells, white cells, or platelets, so that the body cannot respond properly to infection or hemorrhage. It is often fatal. The relation of chloramphenicol to aplastic anemia is discussed further in Chapter 9.

antibiotic." Dr. Watkins gave the drug to his son and testified that it caused his death.[15]

The support of medical journals by advertising is a doubtful blessing. The kinds of medical journals that attract large amounts of advertising, the journals beamed at the practicing physician, are already too numerous to read. Add to these the dozens of "throwaway" journals (those that come free, without request, and are supported entirely by advertisements), and it is obvious that the practicing doctor is overwhelmed with reading material. The conscientious doctor tries to read them all, fearing that if he weakens, he may miss a pearl that the previous journal had failed to gather; the careless or lazy doctor doesn't read even the first journal. It is true that a decrease in the number and size of journals that publish original scientific articles might be harmful, but advertisements for drugs play little part in these. A recent issue of the *Journal of Laboratory and Clinical Medicine*, for instance, contained only one and a half pages of advertisements for therapeutic drugs (plus a one-page advertisement by the Pharmaceutical Manufacturers Association on generic names). The other fifty and a half pages of advertisements were for laboratory apparatus, substances used for diagnostic tests, and books.

Thus, a realistic appraisal of the first claim of the drug industry regarding the value of its promotional practices leads to the conclusion that advertisements may help the physician by reminding him of the advent of new drugs, and by giving him new facts on old drugs promptly, but that this information can come to him in other and better ways. The general informational value of drug advertising is even more questionable and can be brought more effectively to the doctor by journals, medical schools, and medical societies, as will be discussed in a later chapter.

The second point that the drug industry makes is even less plausible: that a doctor does not have to listen to the detail man; he can refuse to see him. He does not have to read the dozen or so advertisements of drugs that come to him unsolicited in the mail in an average day; he can throw them into the wastebasket unopened. To emphasize this point the industry's spokesmen say that the doctor must find these methods of promotion useful because he acts on them. Their marketing surveys show that the success of their advertising campaigns can be measured by the pile of prescriptions on file in the neighborhood drug store. Advertising poor products is self-defeating, the companies contend; the louder they speak out for a poor drug, the more the doctor will remember that it failed. These contentions are a sample of the specious reasoning that characterizes the advertising industry in general. When advertising meets you wherever you turn, it is hard to avoid it; when it is uninhibited by the canons of taste, it can and does push the sedate article in the medical journal into a back seat.

The criticisms of drug advertising have been answered at times by carrying the offensive to the doctors. One writer unmasked a common belief of the advertising expert by charging:

"What these howls of outrage and hurt amount to is that the medical profession is distressed to find its high opinion of itself not shared by writers of ethical drug advertising. It would be a great step forward if doctors stopped bemoaning this attack on their professional maturity and began recognizing how thoroughly justified it is."[16]

He concluded that promotional practices that will not work will not be continued, but that there is no danger of this because, despite the hearings of the Kefauver Committee, "the doctor's pen has not dried up but is flowing more freely than ever." We can answer this cynical comment with another equally cynical. Perhaps the doctor is in the position of the stranger in the small town in the West who was playing in a faro game. When told that the game was crooked, he said he knew that, but it was the only one in town.

Certainly a game that supplies abundant funds to one side to hire the most imaginative propagandists, to purchase pages and pages of slick paper and highly colored print, and to pay out thousands of dollars per year to have a personal representative of a company wait in the doctor's reception room for an hour to spend a few minutes talking with him, while the other side has meager funds and must do its planning in off-hours after an exhausting day of taking care of patients—such a game is one-sided to say the least. Nevertheless, these charges should jolt the medical profession into doing more about the doctor's post-graduate education than it is doing today. For there is enough truth in them to make the doctors wince.

The third defense of the drug industry is a vigorous denial that drug advertising is untruthful, accompanied by the assertion that it is no more misleading than one can expect from the "puffery" that should be allowed in any advertisement. In support of this argument the industry contends that in most companies the medical director or some other physician has the final say on the content and wording of an advertisement. But how significant is this approval? I know many medical directors in industry. They are conscientious, competent, and well-informed about their own drugs and about therapeutics in general. But in the nature of the case they are not free agents. They are em-ployees of a company whose purpose is to make money. Some-times they can resist the combined pressures of the scientist who has devised the drug and takes a personal interest in its success, the director of marketing who wants to put it out tomorrow, and the executive who is worried about the red ink on the balance sheet and looks to the new drugs for salvation. At other times, they must feel that they are

> . . . *a pipe for fortune's finger*
> *To sound what stop she pleases.*

For although the physician in industry is in a strategic position to say no at the right time, it would take a saint to say no for-ever; also, if he says no once too often, he can be fired in a moment, and what other company will hire a man with the reputation of saying no at the wrong time? As I have said before, the relative position of the medical directors has been down-graded in the hierarchy of the pharmaceutical companies in the past few years. That they have done as much as they have is a credit to their intelligence, patience, and heroism. They deserve the strong support of their colleagues in the medical profession, but it is a sad fact that one cannot count on medical directors to reform the drug industry.

Then too, what about the companies that don't give a physician the final word on their advertising? Even the Principles of Ethical Drug Promotion adopted by the Pharmaceutical Manufacturers Association, which is supposed to be an ideal code that all member-companies are expected to follow, does not state that approval of a physician is required for an advertisement but only that "All medical claims and assertions should have medical review prior to their release." "In some companies," Dr. Dale Console told the Kefauver Committee, "the medical director is more or less a screen, and by that I mean a smokescreen. He merely throws a cloak of respectability over what are really business decisions."[17] When the company with a "smokescreen" medical director decides to make a claim for its drugs, what happens to the medical director in a competing company who fulfills his proper function? He will be overruled. "He has one vote," Dr. Console explained. Thus a sort of Gresham's law operates, and bad advertising drives out good.

The fourth defense of the pharmaceutical industry is that the companies advertise as they do because it is good business. The industry's spokesmen claim, for instance, that advertising increases the volume of a drug sold and thus decreases the cost of production. Now this is one of the strong arguments adduced for advertising in general: it has made possible the mass production that in turn has contributed to our prosperity. But is the claim valid when applied to drugs? In the first place, as I have already shown, in many fields there are too many drugs that differ so little that they are practically the same. Instead of twenty-four antihistaminic drugs, we would be better off with five or six and still have enough for vigorous competition. And there are hundreds of mixtures of drugs that have no excuse for being. Like the people in Koko's song, they never would be missed. Conceding that convenience sometimes justifies combining two or perhaps three drugs in a single tablet, there is no reason to combine a half-dozen drugs nor to juggle the proportions of each ingredient so that in the end dozens of permutations and combinations are marketed. The important fact is that if the number of drugs or mixtures were diminished, the volume of those that remained would be increased, and thus the production costs of the remaining drugs would be lowered.

More significant from the standpoint of health, however, is the fact that any attempt to increase the demand for a drug beyond a certain point means that the drug will be given when it isn't needed. Demands for soaps, perfumes, and automobiles can be expanded indefinitely, if people can pay for them; demand for antibiotics, sedatives, and diuretics has a ceiling that is determined by the number of patients who need them. Any attempt to push above that ceiling not only costs more money, but also results in poorer medical care.

One further point with regard to volume. An increase in volume of one drug sold means a decrease in the competitor's drug, unless, as I said before, the drug were to be prescribed when it is not needed. Since Adam Smith's laws do not seem to apply to drug companies (one practically never hears of a company failing in business) because the prices are administered rather than fixed on the basis of costs, the company with the small volume may still be able to sell at a profit even though the costs of manufacture are greater. One must conclude, therefore, that the claim that advertising increases volume and thus reduces costs is a specious one that is improperly transferred from industries where it more legitimately applies.

The claim that advertising increases competition and that competition stirs rival companies to greater efforts cannot be lightly dismissed. Some officials in the Soviet Union are complaining that the drug industry there is not as productive as it should be because there is no advertising.[18] Of course, one must be careful in making comparisons of this kind, since the Soviet industrial economy differs from ours in other respects than the lack of competition. It is newer and has less know-how and fewer trained technicians; furthermore, national policies determine precedence, and some raw materials needed by the pharmaceutical industry may be diverted to defense or construction industries with a higher priority. Nevertheless, competition has undoubtedly helped to keep the quality of drugs produced by some companies in this country at a high level. This kind of a spur may be needed less in the future, however. For example, in a similar comparison between American and Soviet industry, drugs were specifically exempted from the need for competitive promotion because the stimulus for the maintenance of quality need not come from competition, since quality is guaranteed by a government regulatory agency.[19]

An important reason for present advertising practices (which is not brought forward by industry spokesmen) is that innovation requires a steady supply of money over a long run—not for just a few months or a year or two. These funds can be assured if the firm has a monopoly on a product as a result of a patent. But patented products can be imitated, and at any moment the innovating firm may have to share its market with a dozen competitors. A monopoly can be maintained more securely and for a longer time if the company has established a brand name firmly in the minds of the purchasers. This, then, is a main reason for brand names, product differentiation, and the advertising that must be mounted to maintain them. The effect of such monopolies in raising prices will be discussed in the last chapter.

It should be plain to the reader that I do not agree with all of the criticisms regarding the promotion of drugs nor with all of the defenses advanced by the drug industry. Somewhere there is a middle ground. Let us take up again the criticisms in the light of the recent discussion and see what can be done about them.

Many of the criticisms deal with slanting and suggestiveness of advertisements and the important omissions, such as adverse reactions to a drug or references to the medical literature from which the doctor could verify the facts given. The Kefauver-Harris amendments have placed the advertising of drugs for the first time in the hands of the FDA. Furthermore, this agency now has more control over the testing of drugs so that facts will be available for drugs when they are marketed that were not always at hand before. As we shall see in Chapter 11, the new laws and regulations should help take care of the criticisms regarding the content of advertisements.

Inaccurate or misleading statements by detail men will still be a problem, because the FDA cannot monitor conversations as it can review printed pages. Every effort should be made to help detail men develop a sense of professional pride in their vocation. We should consider following the example of France, where the National Syndicate of Pharmaceutical Manufacturers conducts a training program for detail men, at the end of which diplomas are given.[20] Another possibility is for detail men to form their own national organization and to adopt a code of ethics, which could be used to withstand the pressure of a drug company for dishonest detailing.

The more factual and accurate information that the doctor will be receiving in the future should enable him to choose more wisely among the competing products so that the "best man may win," and obviously the poorest ones will drop out of the race. To make the doctor still better informed, however, will require not only the efforts of the FDA but of the medical societies, medical educators, and practicing physicians themselves. The challenge will therefore be up to industry, to government, and to scientists in universities and research institutes to fill the vacuum left by the diminution in the number of "me-too" drugs with truly new drugs. Whether under the new system the costs of advertising will be balanced by what advertising will contribute to the people's health remains to be seen.

The statesmen who framed the U.S. Constitution were very mindful of the need for a careful division of powers and responsibilities within organized society. This resulted in their creation of the delicate balance of power which exists between the executive, legislative, and judicial branches of our Federal Government. In many respects this carefully balanced system . . . closely parallels . . . the present means of supplying safe and effective drugs in the United States.

> —DR. EDWARD G. FELDMANN

No country in the world can match our own in voluntary resources, in voluntary initiative, and in voluntary achievement.

Voluntary-ism has been part of America's genius since the days when Alexis de Toqueville first described us, as a people.

> —SENATOR HUBERT H. HUMPHREY

8

Private Regulation of Drugs:

THE UNITED STATES PHARMACOPEIA and THE NATIONAL FORMULARY

We are accustomed in the United States to thinking that we are governed entirely by local, state, and federal governments, but we forget the large number of quasi-public groups that control people's actions and thus participate in government. These private agencies that assume a public function vary all the way from a local Citizens' Committee or the Friends of the Library to national bodies, such as the American Red Cross and the National Association of Manufacturers. Each affects some of the actions of some of the citizenry and thus complements the actions of the established government. Without these quasi-public organizations, effective government in a democracy would be impossible because it could not penetrate into all the chinks and crevices of men's lives without being prohibitively expensive and unacceptably authoritarian. With them, a democracy functions more extensively and more directly in the interests of the individual citizens.

In the distant past the purchaser of a drug had some means of guessing that a drug was not all it was supposed to be. As the writer of Ecclesiastes said, "Dead flies cause the ointment of the apothecary to send forth a stinking savour." And the buyer could check on the producer directly as did a physician of Alexandria in the first century A.D., when he wrote,

> *Prokleius to his good friend Pekysis, greetings.*
> *You will do well if at your own risk you sell to my*
> *friend Sotas such drugs of good quality as he will*
> *tell you he needs, for him to bring me at Alexandria.*
> *For if you act otherwise and give him rotten stuff,*
> *unsaleable in Alexandria, know that you will have*
> *to deal with me about the cost. Greet all your*
> *family from me. Farewell.*[1]

But as commerce and technology expanded and became more complex, the consumer was progressively less able to judge the merits of what he was buying at the same time that he was receding farther and farther away from the site of manufacture. It was especially important that the drugs he took be checked beforehand because they had such potential for help or harm and because small differences in quantity or potency could produce great changes in the human body.

The technologically advanced countries on the European continent passed laws to regulate the purity and potency of drugs, but in Great Britain, in contrast, inspection of the activities of the apothecaries who prepared and sold the drugs was placed under the Royal College of Physicians. Later the apothecaries formed their own regulatory group, and both groups worked in a parallel manner (and sometimes in opposition) until 1868, when the first major law was passed placing regulation of drugs in the hands of the government.

In the United States the sequence followed the English pattern. Doctors and pharmacists, seeking standards by which to judge the purity and efficacy of drugs, formed the United States Pharmacopeial Convention in 1820. This body set the standards so effectively that, beginning with the 1905 edition, the *USP* (*United States Pharmacopeia*) was recognized by federal laws. The pharmacopeial conventions were composed of representatives from the schools of medicine and pharmacy and the national medical and pharmaceutical associations. Later, in 1888, the American Pharmaceutical Association began to publish the *NF* (*National Formulary*), which set standards for certain drugs not included in the *USP*. The AMA entered the picture with the formation of the Council on Pharmacy and Chemistry in 1905, and the American Dental Association established its Council on Dental Therapeutics in 1930.

Partly because much of the work of regulation was carried on by the private organizations, partly because of inertia, and partly because of resistance to anything that would strengthen the national government (even though state governments were indifferent to the problems or ineffective in solving them), the federal government became involved only gradually. The Biologicals Act of 1902 and the Pure Food and Drugs Act of 1906 were limited in scope and had to be extended by other laws, especially the Food, Drug and Cosmetic Act of 1938 and the Drug Amendments Act of 1962.

In this and the succeeding chapters I shall follow the same sequence, looking first at the activities of private agencies in relation to drugs and then at the actions of the federal and state governments. Finally, the optimal balance between these groups will be considered.

Lists of drugs with formulas of the ingredients were compiled from antiquity, but the invention of printing stimulated the compiling as well as the distribution of such data. The first printed formulary was the *Antidotarium* of Nicolaus Salernitanus, who lived in the twelfth century. It was published in Venice in 1471, one of the earliest medical books printed. By the sixteenth century a number of pharmacopeias had been published in Germany, the most erudite of which was edited by Adolph Occo III and was first published in Augsburg in 1565. By the time the American nation was founded, pharmacopeias were abundant on the European continent. In the British Isles, the London and Edinburgh pharmacopeias had gone through several editions. At the end of the American Revolution the doctors in America relied mostly on these.

The first attempt at a pharmacopeia in the United States was compiled in 1778 for the military hospital in Lititz, Pennsylvania, by Dr. William Brown,[2] physician-general of the medical department of George Washington's army. Although this slender volume met the emergent needs of war, peacetime medicine demanded more.

American doctors were using quite a few drugs made from American plants; they wanted these included. Other complaints were later summed up in the preface to the first edition of the *USP*. Doctors objected to "the evil of irregularity and uncertainty in the preparation of medicine." They wanted the older pharmacopeias pruned of little-used drugs, contending that "the fault of the lists of the *Materia Medica* which have been adopted in different countries, has always been their redundancy rather than their deficiency. The number of articles necessary for the management of diseases . . . is always very far short of the catalogue afforded by most Pharmacopeias." Finally, they complained of the variety and complexity of names that were given to drugs: "The essential properties of names ought to be expressiveness, brevity and dissimilarity."[3]

The Massachusetts Medical Society attempted to remedy these deficiencies when it published a pharmacopcia in 1808. But since this and the other local pharmacopeias that followed were based on the pharmacopeias of the Old World, they did not represent the consensus of the American medical practice. Pressure for a truly national compendium continued to build up. As a result delegates from medical societies of the Eastern cities met on January 1, 1820, in the Senate chamber in Washington and prepared an initial draft of what was to become the first edition of the USP. Its object was stated in the preface to be: "to select from among substances which possess medicinal power, those, the utility of which is most fully established and best understood; and to form from them preparations and compositions, in which their powers may be exerted to the greatest advantage."[4]

Thus the modern concept of a pharmacopeia is a compendium that contains only the most approved drugs and sets standards to assure that they will be optimally prepared. These principles have been adhered to in the successive revisions.

From the start, the USP has been governed by democratic processes. Soon after the first edition was published, a call went out to all medical societies and medical schools of the country for a pharmacopeial convention to be held in 1830. This and subsequent meetings every decade have determined the rules under which successive editions have been prepared.

As schools of pharmacy were founded and pharmaceutical societies were formed, they were invited to take part and were given full membership in the Pharmacopeial Convention by 1850. Since the USP served the pharmacists' needs especially, the representatives of this profession plunged energetically into the work—so much so that by 1900, in the face of waning support from the medical profession, the pharmacists had practically taken over the work of revision. Dr. E. R. Squibb, the founder of the pharmaceutical company of that name, tried to prod physicians into an interest in the *USP* with indifferent success. But by 1910 the ferment of reform in medical education was beginning to stimulate a more scientific approach toward drugs, and from 1920 on, physicians increasingly supported the *USP*. Representatives from the federal government were added in the 1830 convention in the persons of the surgeon-general of the army, the senior surgeon of the navy, and the members of Congress who were physicians. The latter were subsequently dropped, but after the *USP* was made a legal standard in 1906, representatives from federal agencies directly involved in the regulation of drugs were increasingly invited to take part. In the 1890 convention, the AMA and the American Pharmaceutical Association were added to the list, followed later by other national societies.

Today the Pharmacopeial Conventions are composed of representatives from the schools and the state societies of medicine and pharmacy plus a number of national societies and government agencies in the health areas. For the last Pharmacopeial Convention, held in 1960, invitations were extended to the 79 colleges of medicine and the 76 colleges of pharmacy, 7 agencies of the federal government, the state medical and pharmaceutical associations, and 12 national professional associations in medicine and pharmacy. Of the 277 groups entitled to representation, 194 sent delegates.

In 1840 a Committee on Revision was appointed for the first time. This has functioned ever since to determine the content of the successive volumes of the *USP*. Today this committee is composed of twenty physicians, approximately twenty pharmacists, and about twenty other scientists. The physicians select the drugs that will be included in the next edition, and the pharmacists determine the standards for those drugs and specify the tests that are to be used to establish their identity and purity. Thus it can be seen that the Pharmacopeial Convention is a democratic association with a wide representation from the interested professional fields and that the responsibility for the compendium is placed in the hands of experts from those fields.

The policies of the organization have followed closely upon

its original purpose, although technological advances have necessitated many changes in approach and procedure. These changes are best considered by reviewing various landmark decisions as they occurred.

In the decade beginning in 1880, the increase in the number of new drugs and the rise of the large-scale drug industry made it imperative to publish in the *USP* for the first time tests and assays to set standards of strength and purity of drugs. This was first done in *USP* VI, published in 1882, and in successive editions the *USP* became a book of authoritative standards.

In 1906 the first comprehensive federal Pure Food and Drugs Act stated that the *USP* and its companion, the *NF*, were official compendia for purposes of determining standards of drugs. Such a delegation of a governmental function to a private agency is unique. It is a tribute to the integrity and expertise of those who determine *USP* policies and an acknowledgment of the worth of what they have produced. In spite of critics who wonder even today how this delegation of powers can be justified,[5] the law that made the *USP* an official compendium was upheld by the Supreme Court of Wisconsin in 1953. Moreover, the legal position of the federal government is protected by a provision in the regulatory act stating that the secretary of Health, Education and Welfare must call attention to the publishers of the *USP* and the *NF* when their standards for a particular drug are not adequate. Because of the efficiency of the two organizations involved, it has not been necessary for the government to invoke this privilege.

Decisions as to which drugs should be admitted to the *USP* were becoming increasingly more difficult as effective drugs were being produced in ever larger numbers. To meet this challenge, a Subcommittee on Scope was formed in 1920. In the decade of the 1930's, a series of articles was sponsored in *The Journal of the American Medical Association* to acquaint physicians with the work and worth of the *USP*. For some reason, this first serious attempt at making the convention an informational agency for physicians as well as for pharmacists died a'borning.

To cope with the rising tide of drugs, formally organized

advisory groups were appointed in 1935 to assist the Committee on Revision. Panels of experts in various therapeutic fields were first used for the fifteenth edition, published in 1955. The 1940 convention voted to publish the *USP* at five-year intervals instead of every decade as before. Also, by 1940 the convention began to prepare and distribute reference standards for a number of drugs in the *USP* that were assayed in animals. (A reference standard is a sample of a drug, usually highly purified, from which portions are taken for comparison with other preparations of the drug that are being tested for identity, quantity, potency, and purity.) This enterprise has increased progressively until today the sale of reference standards brings in half of the income of the organization.

In 1960 a new section was added, entitled "Adjuncts and Clinical Reagents." This set standards for substances that were used in the laboratory rather than in the human body but that were added to the *USP* because their results would affect the diagnosis, prevention, or treatment of disease in humans.

Thus, in several ways the *USP* widened its scope to keep up with the expanding field of therapy and stepped up its pace to keep abreast of advances in discovery. But a contrary trend can also be seen. Beginning in 1941 the federal government began to encroach on the hitherto private preserves of the *USP*. In that year the FDA was charged with certifying each batch of insulin produced. This action was taken because the patent on insulin was expiring and it was feared that uniformity of effectiveness would be lost in diversity of manufacture. Since even a small variation in potency might mean the difference between life and death in a diabetic patient, it seemed imperative to have individual batches tested by the government before they were marketed. In 1945 the process of testing individual batches and certification was extended to include a few antibiotics and in the 1962 act, over the protests of the *USP*, to cover all of them.

From its inception the *USP* had selected a name for each drug adopted for inclusion, which became the "official" nonproprietary or generic name of the drug. If the drug had been previously included in the AMA's *New and Nonofficial Remedies* (*NNR*), later *New and Nonofficial Drugs* (*NND*), the name used therein was usually selected. Also the *USP* consulted the manufacturer of the drug and the private and official groups in other countries who were involved in naming drugs, but it reserved the right to make the final decision. Beginning in 1961 representatives of the *USP* and the AMA began to select names jointly. In 1964 a representative of the *NF* was added, and finally, in 1967, a member of the staff of the FDA. The nomenclature of drugs will be discussed further in Chapter 9.

As might have been expected in an expanding field, people within the pharmacopeial committees and without have wanted the *USP* to do more things than it has done. The *USP* has served primarily as a book of standards by which to measure what a drug is, whether it is pure, and whether it has the strength (potency) it is said to have. It has performed this function well. It has thus served the needs of the drug-makers, the regulatory agencies, and to a certain extent the pharmacists. For the practicing physician, on the other hand, it has had little significance. Toward the end of the nineteenth and the beginning of the twentieth century, when drugs and mixtures of varying strengths were freely marketed, the initials "USP" came to mean a drug that the physician could depend upon as having uniform potency; he knew that the effect a given dose would produce could be matched by a similar dose in the same or another patient. But as federal laws required all drugs to conform to established standards and as the flood of new drugs with attractive trademark (brand) names captured his attention, the physician came to take proper standardization for granted. The initials "USP" disappeared from advertisements, and the physician no longer looked for them.

Likewise abortive attempts have been made from time to time to establish the *USP* as a therapeutic guide for the physician. Selection of drugs for a pharmacopeia could be made according to either of two criteria: how frequently they are prescribed, or their value compared to other drugs available on the market as determined by expert and knowledgeable physicians in each field of therapy. Admission of drugs to the *USP* has been mostly by the latter criterion, but extent of use has had its influence, sometimes to a greater and sometimes to a lesser extent. For example, over thirty chemically different antihistaminic drugs are sold today (plus many combinations with other drugs). They all have some effectiveness; they all have some adverse reactions. If they were all listed in the *USP* it would become a mere inventory of the drugs available; on the other hand, choosing only one of them would not afford the opportunity for a substitution in the case of the patient who has an adverse reaction to that drug. In the 1965 edition of the *USP* the Subcommittee on Scope compromised by listing five antihistaminics. In general, when there was no clear superiority with respect to effectiveness or adverse reactions among drugs of similar chemical structure, the committee gave preference to the first drug marketed. Thus, the *USP* does represent a "blue ribbon list" of drugs by which a physician could practice high quality medicine, seldom, if ever, having to resort to a nonpharmacopeial drug. Why then is it not so used?

First, doctors cherish the idea that they are independent and want to feel that they can use whatever drugs they please—a flame that is fanned by every pharmaceutical company that would like to sell more of its products (and what company wouldn't?). Second, new drugs appear after the list has been decided upon for each five-year edition. This hiatus is partly filled by the publication of supplements, but there is always a time lag because after the drugs have been agreed upon, several months are needed for the establishment of standards of purity and efficacy. In a survey of drugs prescribed in one city in 1964, 32 per cent of the items were listed in the *USP*, 20 per cent in the *NF*, and 48 per cent in neither.[6]

Finally, the *USP* fails as a therapeutic guide for the physician because he finds nothing in it to help him except the name of the drug, its general therapeutic class, and the usual dose-range. The book serves mainly the manufacturer and the regulatory official. It is rarely seen on the physician's bookshelf.

Perhaps the *USP* could be made so valuable to the practicing physician that he would buy it and use it if therapeutic information would be added, but this would make the book too large and unwieldy. The unique contribution of the *USP* to the physician is the careful winnowing out of the most valuable drugs from the chaff of the "me-too" drugs, a procedure that occupies hours and days of effort by some of the nation's top experts. Added to this are the decisions on the proper dosages of the drugs admitted to the *USP*. A separate volume on therapy incorporating this information could be the *vade mecum* of the practicing physician. In the past the AMA attempted this by publishing the *Epitome of the United States Pharmacopeia and the National Formulary*, but abandoned it after several editions. Its publication and distribution were never an important objective of the Council on Pharmacy and Chemistry; perhaps this is the reason why it was never widely used. If the Pharmacopeial Convention had chosen to use its facilities to publish a book on therapy as a companion to the USP and had publicized it widely, it might have done for therapy what William Osler's textbook did for the understanding and diagnosis of disease by practicing doctors at the turn of the century. Certainly no book has yet appeared to fill that function. The void may be filled by the book that the Council on Drugs is now preparing, *AMA Drug Evaluations* (*ADE*). (See Chapter 9.)

In another area the *USP* has hesitated to move ahead. When pressure for the regulation of drug standards first reached the point where some organized efforts were made, doctors and pharmacists were forced to direct their efforts to areas where technological change had made establishment of standards possible. As a consequence, chemical standards for identity and purity were developed gradually over the course of a few decades. Biological assay, the testing of the effect of a drug on an intact animal or upon the organs of an animal, followed soon after, and both methods were extended and improved as new classes of drugs were introduced and new instruments of measurement were devised by chemists and biologists. What a drug did in man was harder to measure because the number of variables to be considered was greater and because the techniques of clinical investigation had not been developed commensurately. Doctors, pharmacists, and regulators slipped into the habit of assuming that if a capsule, tablet, elixir, or ampule contained the proper amount of a sufficiently pure drug, the drug would have the predicted effect upon a patient. Only recently, when proponents of prescribing by trade names began to dispute with advocates of prescribing by generic names, have we been forced to look at the differences between drugs that contain identical amounts of a therapeutically active substance.

One obvious way to find out whether different preparations of a particular drug are equally effective is to try each one on a number of normal persons and measure the physiologic response, or to test each preparation in patients to see whether it shortens the illness or abates the symptoms. But this would be a Herculean task that might well involve the entire medical profession in testing and the entire population as subjects of the tests.

The simplest test would be to measure the speed with which each preparation goes into solution, either with or without agitation. Studies now in progress may produce tests for many drugs that would correlate closely with their therapeutic effects.

For other drugs it will undoubtedly be necessary to rely on a test that measures more closely what happens in the human body. This is the determination of the quantity of the drug present in the blood after ingestion, which should be a good measure of the availability of the drug in the organs where it acts (often called physiologic or biologic availability). As of today, techniques have not been devised for making these measurements for all drugs, but methods have been perfected for enough to occupy us for some time; meanwhile we can devise techniques for other drugs.

The *USP* and the *NF* recently established a Joint Panel on Physiologic Availability.[7] Since the FDA is being prodded by congressional critics into making decisions with respect to physiologic availability, it is imperative for the private regulatory groups to move rapidly if they do not want to see one more area slip completely under governmental control. From the standpoint of the government agencies, it would seem reasonable that if effective standards could be set up by authoritative sources like the *USP* and the *NF*, the FDA could bend its efforts to applying those standards and be relieved of the task of making them, as has been true of chemical tests and biological assays. This will be discussed further in Chapter 11.

Another vacuum into which the *USP* could move, if it wishes, is the field of drug mixtures. In the days when most drugs were worthless, it mattered little whether a prescription listed a single ingredient or a score of them. One famous preparation, called theriac, which lingered on in France until the beginning of the twentieth century, contained as many as seventy-one different substances. As modern knowledge of chemistry, physiology, and clinical medicine enabled doctors to pinpoint and quantify the actions of drugs, the worthless ones were eliminated and doctors prescribed single remedies more frequently. The best doctors today seldom prescribe combinations of drugs, except for the convenience or comfort of the patient. But some doctors' habits have not kept pace with advancing knowledge, and hundreds of mixtures are on the market and are being prescribed. With the exception of a few, which are honored by long usage, none is listed today in the *USP*. The ignoring of mixtures by the *USP* had much to do with the establishment of the other official compendium, which will be discussed next.

Soon after the pharmacists founded their national society, the American Pharmaceutical Association, in the mid-nineteenth century, pressure began to build up for a publication that would list standards for drugs that doctors were prescribing but which were not listed in the *USP*. Among these were many mixtures. To meet these needs the American Pharmaceutical Association published the first edition of the *NF* in 1888. It established standards for 435 mixtures. As successive editions appeared, at first irregularly and later at ten- and five-year intervals, following the publication of each edition of the *USP*, the percentage of mixtures declined and the proportion of single drugs increased. This was augmented by the practice of accepting for the *NF* the drugs that were discarded from the *USP*, except for those that were prescribed so seldom that they could be dropped from both compendia. The last edition of the *NF* contained only about twenty-five monographs on combinations out of a total of approximately eight hundred monographs. Mixtures are now selected for the *NF* only if the combination provides some therapeutic advantage over the administration of the individual drugs.[8] Since practically none are listed in the *USP*, it is apparent that neither of the official compendia attempts to set standards for the majority of the mixtures sold and prescribed today.

The *NF* fulfilled an important need and soon paid its own way. In 1917 the American Pharmaceutical Association set aside the income from the *NF* in a separate fund so that the profits of the enterprise could be used for research to develop new standards for drugs. At present the *NF* is published by the National Formulary Board, which is composed of the director of the National Formulary, a secretary, and nine members elected by the Board of Trustees of the American Pharmaceutical Association. The responsibility for selection of drugs rests upon a Committee on Admissions of twenty members, seventeen of whom are physicians or pharmacologists. Standards are established by a Committee on Specifications of fifty members representing the pharmaceutical, chemical, and biological sciences. The board gives final approval to the actions of both committees.

Another activity of the National Formulary Board is the development of reference standards for drugs listed in the *NF*, which are then sold to interested parties for use in conducting laboratory tests. The American Pharmaceutical Association also houses a Drug Standards Laboratory for the chemical testing of drugs. Since 1961, when the AMA and the United States Pharmacopeial Convention each undertook to provide one third of the financial support, this laboratory has been called the American Pharmaceutical Association Foundation Drug Standards Laboratory.

In 1930 the *NF* pioneered by making a survey to determine how often doctors prescribed the drugs in its previous edition and other drugs that were not included in either the *USP* or the *NF*. Also studied at the same time was the number of prescriptions compounded in drugstores throughout the United States, as compared with those that were merely dispensed as prepared by the manufacturer. A later survey in cooperation with the

United States Bureau of the Census covered 121,924 prescriptions written during 1930 and 1931.⁹

The National Formulary Board has used such surveys to help it decide which drugs would be included in the *NF*. In recent years, however, it has been even more selective and in 1961 formally revised its policy so as to admit drugs solely on the basis of therapeutic value. Thus it is now following the path that the *USP* has been taking since its inception. If this trend continues, why do we need two books and two sets of selection committees? Cannot the *USP* and the *NF* be combined? The two books use similar methods of establishing standards and, by definite agreement, identical editorial policies. As the Director of the National Formulary has testified, aside from the drugs admitted, the two books are virtually identical.¹⁰ If the historical accidents that created them separately are to be justified in subsequent editions, it is imperative for the *USP* to establish its selective status by promulgating a list of the most valuable drugs that the doctor can use in practice, for it must somehow influence the doctor to practice according to that list.

Better still would be a merger of the *USP* and the *NF*, along with a system of classifying the drugs of primary importance, those less significant, and those that had not been adequately tested as yet. The significant and the much-used mixtures should also be included and classified in the same way. My recommendations for providing doctors with an up-to-date list of drugs, their properties, and their uses will be given in Chapter 11.

9

Private Regulation of Drugs (Continued):

THE AMERICAN MEDICAL ASSOCIATION and THE AMERICAN DENTAL ASSOCIATION

O f all the private agencies in America, the AMA has worked the hardest to see that drugs are safe and effective and that the claims made for them are reasonable and accurate. The activities of the AMA in the field of drugs fall into three periods, which I have called anticipatory, regulatory, and educational. The first extended from the formation of the AMA in 1847 to the establishment of its Council on Pharmacy and Chemistry in 1905; the second from 1905 until 1955, when the Seal of Acceptance program was dropped; and the third from 1955 to the present.

THE ANTICIPATORY PERIOD. Although the preamble of the AMA constitution written in 1847 contained nothing closer to therapeutics than that the association was formed "for cultivating and advancing medical knowledge,"[1] agitation from the state medical societies for some control of drugs began early. At the first annual meeting in 1848 a resolution was introduced requesting that a committee be appointed to standardize anesthetics. In the subsequent years many voices protested the "quack remedies . . . now palmed upon the public" and emphasized the need for doctors to know exactly what these nostrums contained. Many doctors resented the shameless advertising of the vendors of these preparations, as well as the glowing testimonials contributed by some of their colleagues.

The Journal of the American Medical Association came in for its share of criticism. One physician in 1883 complained that the drugs it advertised were no better than quack medicines. A few attempts were made to rid the journal of the worst of the advertisements; in 1884 the Board of Trustees reported that a regulation restricting advertising, which had been adopted at the 1880 meeting, "was a wise restraint tending to elevate the dignity of The Journal but at the same time deprive it of a considerable revenue." Thus popped out into the open a dilemma which has plagued the AMA ever since. When in 1892 the Philadelphia

County Medical Society asked that *The Journal of the American Medical Association* eliminate proprietary advertisements altogether, the editor defended the practice because the journal could not afford the loss of revenue and doctors were "prescribing greater amounts of these preparations." Nevertheless, the policy was tightened the next year when a Committee on Advertising was formed to pass on advertisements referred by the editor. At the same time manufacturers were required to submit the complete formulas of their preparations.[2]

In spite of the improvements in advertisements, the tempo of protest rose in the early years of the century. At the same time reforms were being pushed in other fields; the AMA itself had launched a campaign for reform in medical education. This produced a report in 1904 on medical education in the United States, which in turn precipitated the formation of the Council on Medical Education. Furthermore, this was the era of muckrakers, and their influence seemed to be felt among the doctors.

In 1900 the editor of the *Cleveland Journal of Medicine* wrote of medical journals: "The greed for advertising patronage leads the editor only too often to prostitute his pen or his pages to the advertiser, so long as he can secure the coveted revenue. So our journals are filled with articles and editorials containing covert advertisements of this and that remedy." As a result of this and similar protests, the wheels began to move. In 1900 a series of articles was begun in the journal "designed to correct the abuses from advertising and patronizing unscientific pharmaceutic preparations."[3] In the 1903 and 1904 annual meetings of the AMA resolutions were introduced requesting the formation of an organization to analyze drugs and examine the claims made for them. Finally, at the 1905 meeting, the Board of Trustees announced that the Council on Pharmacy and Chemistry had been organized on February 11 of that year (Table 7).

THE REGULATORY PERIOD. A strong council was appointed at the start. It was composed of six professors from schools of medicine, four from schools of pharmacy, and three members from the

TABLE 7. Important Dates in the AMA's Programs on Drugs

Program	Begun	Ended
Council on Pharmacy and Chemistry	1905	1956
Council on Drugs	1956	
New and Nonofficial Remedies published	1907	1957
New and Nonofficial Drugs published	1958	1964
New Drugs published	1965	
Useful Drugs published	1913	1952
Seal of Acceptance Program	1930	1955
Committee on Blood Dyscrasias	1953	1960
Committee on Adverse Reactions	1960	
Registry of Adverse Reactions	1963	
AMA-USP Committee on Nomenclature	1961	1964
United States Adopted Names Council	1964	

federal government—one from the Public Health Service and two from the Department of Agriculture. One of the latter was that militant champion of the consumer Harvey W. Wiley, whose passion for reform will be discussed in more detail in the next chapter. No less a crusader was the chairman of the council, George H. Simmons, secretary and general manager of the AMA and able editor of its journal.

The council immediately adopted rules governing the admission of drugs to their official publication, *NNR* (*New and Nonofficial Remedies*), rules that sound very modern today. These required that the identity, ingredients, strength, and proof of purity of all drugs be provided, that the drug should not be advertised to the public, that labeling should not be false or misleading, and that advertising should not be exaggerated or misleading. The rules also provided that the council might select a name for the drug if the name used was objectionable.[4]

The vigorous policies of the council brought anguished cries from some drug manufacturers and counterattacks from others. The editor stated in 1906 that the enemies of the AMA's policy included the Proprietary Association of America, the so-called "ethical" proprietary medicine makers whose products did not bear inspection, and privately owned medical journals more or less dependent upon these two groups for their income. The attacks during this period reached the acme of viciousness, including smears on Simmons's private life. "Caricature, ridicule, invective, misrepresentation, half statements, and distortions of the truth have all been utilized to check the work of the Association," cried the editor of the journal.[5]

One firm, the M. J. Breitenbach Company, threatened to withdraw its advertising from the journal because of an editorial warning doctors against "blind reliance" on iron and quinine in the treatment of anemias. This company, with a mixture of naïveté and effrontery, contended that advertisements in the journal should be "taken into consideration" when an editorial was written.[6]

It is well to note parenthetically that the crusading zeal of the AMA in the drug battle at this time was matched by zeal in other areas. It was a strong advocate of food and drug regulatory bills that had been introduced into Congress for several years before the passage of the first act in 1906; it vigorously supported state laws that had the same objectives; it ruthlessly exposed the numerous quacks who were preying upon the public's health and pocketbook; it attacked the newspapers for not publicizing convictions of "large and respected" drug firms for misbranding and adulterating food and drugs. Also at this time (1910) its House of Delegates authorized for the first time the publication of ratings of medical schools into Group A, B, or C on the basis of their facilities, faculty, and standards.[7]

The activities of the Council on Pharmacy and Chemistry brought on some bitter fights. After a prolonged legal battle with the makers of "Wine of Cardui," which the council called "disguised booze," the court ruled in favor of the drug company, chiefly because the editor of the journal had made much of the company president's high position in the Methodist Church, but the damages were only one cent and the AMA considered it had won a moral victory.[8]

Thus, an editorial in the journal in 1915 could report triumphantly: "Habit-forming and other dangerous drugs are far less common in the nostrums than they were ten years ago." Nevertheless it mentioned one preparation that was recommended for the treatment of alcoholism and for the preparation of highballs on the same label.[9] Further evidence of the success of the council's fight was a new rule added in 1924 that the council would refuse admission of a drug to AMA publications if the firm making the drug marketed a large proportion of its products without council approval.[10]

In the 1920's the council stated that the "complex mixtures of simple drugs exploited to our profession under fanciful names and with extravagant claims" had been forced into obscurity, but that "worthless vaccine and endocrine products made from crude extracts of many organs and dangerous intravenous preparations had taken their place."[11] The council declared war against all three and kept up a steady barrage of articles, speeches, and reports against them, while denying the makers advertising space in the AMA journals. The campaign gradually won the respect of most of the practicing physicians, although, sad to relate, some continued to be seduced by the advertiser's wiles or duped by their own stupidity, even as some still are today.

On the scientific side, the council's Committee on Therapeutic Research, which had been formed in 1912, continued to finance research on therapy with sums that, although extremely modest by today's standards, were sufficient to meet significant needs at that time. The council also co-operated in the early clinical trials of the anesthetic ethylene[12] and surveyed the administration of barbiturates among 1,125,000 patients in hospitals, concluding that addiction to barbiturates was common "and the promiscuous use of these preparations is clearly responsible for many accidental intoxications that have produced fatal results."[13] The council also published a detailed and thoughtful report on the cost of clinical research, to guide clinicians who were desirous of investigating drugs.[14]

In the decade before 1955 the Therapeutics Trials Committee seems to have been especially active, sponsoring investigations of such diverse treatments as moist heat in poliomyelitis, chlorophyll in wound healing, the aluminum treatment of silicosis, streptomycin in granuloma inguinale, methyl cellulose in constipation, and the steroid hormones in cancer of the breast.[15]

That the work of the council had the endorsement of the AMA

is apparent from numerous laudatory reports by the Board of Trustees. Also, the presidential address of Dr. Herman Kretschmer in 1944 complained that of five thousand prescriptions filled by Chicago drugstores, only 62 per cent had been for drugs in the official compendiums and in *NNR*, whereas 27 per cent had been for proprietary remedies and 11 per cent for vitamins.[16] He called this a "sad state of affairs" and implored teachers in medical schools and practitioners to "follow the statements of the Council on Pharmacy and Chemistry," stressing the fact that "use of such agents in preference to proprietary drugs will permit savings of thousands of dollars." In 1946 the Board of Trustees noted that "the Council's office has been swamped with presentations of products from firms that are now striving to bring their policies into conformance with Council principles as well as from already recognized manufacturers. . . ."[17]

The pharmaceutical industry had some criticisms, but they were mostly constructive. In a conference called by the council in 1946 the drug firms suggested that the council evaluate mixtures as well as single drugs, that it speed up its evaluations, and that it exempt certain *USP* articles from consideration. In 1947 the American Pharmaceutical Manufacturers Association gave its scientific award to the AMA "in recognition of the services which were rendered in behalf of service to the public and medical research."[18] And in 1953 the director of clinical research for one of the larger pharmaceutical companies wrote: "Although at times manufacturers may experience delays or adverse decisions of the Council on Pharmacy and Chemistry, no one desires to discontinue this function of the American Medical Association. On the contrary, we cherish the right of a nongovernmental and extralegal group of physicians to make public their judgments about the products of pharmaceutical industry. The Council has been an important factor in the progress of American drug production."[19]

As late as 1954 the council's program seemed to be meeting with approval, for the Board of Trustees reported that for the year September 1, 1953, to September 1, 1954, 223 products had been submitted for acceptance and that "apparently most pharmaceutical firms were not reluctant to have their worthwhile new products evaluated by an independent group of experts in the field of drug therapy."[20]

And then, in 1955, came an abrupt shift in policy, the dropping of the Seal of Acceptance program. Before analyzing the reasons for this change, let us take a look at the attitude of the AMA toward the advertising of drugs during the regulatory era.

In announcing the formation of the Council on Pharmacy and Chemistry, the Board of Trustees stated: "The subject of ethical advertising has been before the Board at practically all of its meetings and has always been both a vexed and an unsolvable one."[21] From the beginning this council was intimately involved with advertising because it set up the criteria by which advertisements were judged, and after 1930 its Seal of Acceptance was the only entrance ticket to the journal's advertising columns. The position of the AMA was strengthened in 1913 by the formation of the Bureau of State Journals, which arranged for screening, in accordance with the concepts of the Council on Pharmacy and Chemistry, of advertisements for journals of the state medical societies that were members (and this at one time included nearly all of the state societies). The same rules applied to the specialty journals published by the AMA and to its monthly magazine for laymen, called *Hygeia* (later *Today's Health*). The AMA's hand was also strengthened by parallel programs for foods and devices run by the Council on Foods and Nutrition and the Council on Physical Medicine.

From 1906 to 1955 an advertising committee was in existence, of which the editor of the journal was chairman. In actuality, the secretary of the Council on Pharmacy and Chemistry examined all advertisements submitted and either rejected them or advised rewriting if the claims did not exceed those considered acceptable by the council. His decisions were almost always agreed upon by the advertising committee, but in the case of a disagreement the final decision rested with the editor, who was also a member of the Council on Pharmacy and Chemistry.

Gradually, the outright quacks and the fringe operators were forced out of the columns of the journal and sometimes out of business, too. The leading companies swung around to a conformity that, even though grudging, nevertheless resulted in better quality products and more realistic statements about them. The shift in attitude of the pharmaceutical companies is illustrated by the change in tenor of the editorials and the reports of the council that appeared in the journal. In 1910 the editor complained that "two directly related interests—the so-called ethical proprietary business and the 'patent medicine' business—by fair means and foul have done their best to discredit and injure the Association."[22] And in 1912 the Board of Trustees in their report regretted that the Council on Pharmacy and Chemistry did not have greater cooperation from the leading pharmaceutical houses of the country.[23]

In contrast, in its 1926 report, the Board of Trustees exulted: "It is gratifying to note that, though careful censorship of advertising material has been maintained, there has been less friction between the Department and those who would use the advertising pages of *The Journal* than in former years."[24]

Another sign that marked a turn in the tide was that, in 1919, receipts from advertising passed the receipts from subscriptions to the AMA journals.[25]

In 1934 the council felt secure enough to add its famous Rule 11, which stated that no products would be accepted by the council from firms whose general promotional practices were unacceptable. Thus at one stroke it greatly expanded the scope of its enforcement. Yet, despite added restrictions, the number of drugs submitted to the council for consideration continued to increase.

The top officials of the Association were behind the movement. In 1939 President Rock Sleyster said, "Today, not only the greatest medical journal in the world, but the state journals and many independent journals show by their clean advertising the imprint of the Council's efforts in furthering rational therapy and enhancing scientific treatment of the sick."[26] And in 1948 Austin Smith, the secretary of the Council on Pharmacy and Chemistry, wrote with regard to advertising, "Never once did any official of the Association attempt to make the Council deviate from the decisions it believed warranted."[27]

It has been noted that in 1919 the receipts from advertising exceeded for the first time the receipts from subscriptions. This flourishing state of affairs continued through the 1930's, but after this, advertising revenue fell behind. In 1949 income from membership dues and subscriptions, $4,817,000, was far ahead of receipts from advertising, which were only $2,432,000. By 1954, the last year of the Seal of Acceptance program, advertising revenue had risen to $3,758,000, but it still had not reached the level of other income, which was about the same as five years before.[28] Whether this relative deficiency in advertising revenue spurred the AMA to drop the Seal of Acceptance program is a disputed question, which we will take up later. First, let us follow the history of the council through the succeeding era.

THE EDUCATIONAL PERIOD. For a few years, the composition of the Council on Pharmacy and Chemistry continued very much as before. Dr. Simmons had remained chairman of the Council through 1927, although by that time he was editor emeritus of *The Journal of the American Medical Association*. He had been succeeded by Dr. Reid Hunt, professor of pharmacology at Harvard. During these years Dr. Torald Sollmann had been vice-chairman. The latter became chairman in 1938 and remained at that post through 1960. The federal government was represented by two officers of the Public Health Service and an official of the FDA.

In 1956 the name of the council was changed to the Council on Drugs, and in 1961 it was given a "new look." Dr. Sollmann, who had been on the council ever since it started, was removed, as were the representatives from the federal government. Dr. Morris Fishbein, who had been a member while editor of the journal, had remained on the council, although no longer on the staff of the AMA, through 1953. When Dr. Austin Smith became editor of the journal, he left the council, and his successor, Dr. Robert Stormont, became the first secretary who was not a member of the council. Thus, by 1960 the staff of the AMA and the federal government were simultaneously shut out from membership. This policy has continued to the present day.

New rules prevented council members from serving longer than ten years and chairman from holding that position for longer than three. While the motive behind these rules was excellent—it was undoubtedly important to get new blood into the councils—the net effect was that the Council on Drugs steered a shifting course for the next few years.

NNR was renamed *New and Nonofficial Drugs* (*NND*) when the name of the council was changed to the Council on Drugs in 1956, but still doctors didn't read it. Finally, in 1964 it was changed drastically to suit the clinician rather than the pharmacologist and named *New Drugs*; its publications and promotion were taken over by the AMA itself. This helped, but still only 31,250 copies were sold in the peak year, 1966, and in 1967 sales dropped off to 19,950.[29]

The council announced an "expanded program" in 1955.[30] It promised evaluation of new drugs or new uses for old drugs at the "earliest possible opportunity" and stated that this information would be published as monographs in *The Journal of the American Medical Association*. The activities of the council under the new program consisted of gathering, evaluating, and disseminating information about drugs.

Pharmaceutical companies were asked to submit data on new drugs simultaneously to the AMA and the FDA. Since the companies were no longer required to gain the Seal of Acceptance in order to advertise, however, the council's teeth were gone. From 1955 until 1962, when the New Drug Amendments Act was passed, the council struggled manfully to persuade drug firms to supply this information. Some complied with the requests; others ignored them. To supplement the information supplied by drug companies or to fill the void when nothing was forthcoming, the staff of the Department of Drugs searched the medical literature and wrote a preliminary monograph. This was sent to consultants, investigators in the field covered by the drug, who may or may not have used the drug themselves, who made their suggestions. Finally, the monograph was revised by a referee, sent to the council members for their opinions, further revised by the staff and the referee, whose decision was final, and published. All of this took many hours of work on the part of the staff, which were reflected in the increased appropriations to the Department of Drugs. Senator Kefauver had made much of the fact that the appropriations to the council fell from $155,000 a year in 1954 to $99,000 in 1956 and $75,000 in 1958, while appropriations for the Department of Public Relations had gone steadily upward during the same period.[31] In retrospect, this appears to have been caused by uncertainty on the part of the council as to the projects it wanted to undertake, the necessary tooling up for new programs, and rapid turnover in the staff of the Department of Drugs. Once the programs were decided upon and leadership was provided, the council's work began moving ahead, as shown by the increase in appropriations for the Department of Drugs to nearly $734,000 by 1968.

Since the Drug Amendments Act of 1962 has been in effect, drug companies have sent data on new drugs to the AMA more rapidly. Whether or not this is because they hope the council will take a favorable look at their drugs and thus provide them with talking points if the FDA delays approval, this change certainly facilitates the work of the council.

One area in which information was glaringly deficient was on adverse reactions to drugs. In 1953 the concern of a number of hematologists and especialy Dr. Maxwell Wintrobe over the aplastic anemias that had appeared in some patients receiving chloramphenicol led to the formation of a Committee on Blood Dyscrasias, and in 1960 this committee was broadened into a Committee on Adverse Reactions. Under its guidance, a Registry on Adverse Reactions was set up for the reporting by physicians in private practice and in hospitals of untoward effects accompanying the administration of drugs. The program attracted much attention, resulted in a number of reports being sent to the Council on Drugs, and provided information which made possible several articles on the deleterious actions of drugs.[32]

Yet the method of collecting data had serious defects. Physicians reported only a small fraction of all cases. Whether this paucity of reports resulted from inertia, or from fear of colleagues' criticism or of malpractice suits cannot be determined; all three probably played a part. A second defect was that the total number of patients receiving a drug was unknown; if the numerator of the ratio was defective, the denominator was entirely absent! Finally, the system did not serve as an early warning system. In no instance was an adverse reaction to a drug reported that had not already been observed elsewhere. This verified a phenomenon that had been observed before: physicians seldom take note of adverse reactions unless they are warned what to look for.

Despite the method of reporting, the Registry on Adverse Reactions was able to demonstrate that certain drugs unquestionably produce adverse reactions. Chloramphenicol is a good example. A tabulation of reports by practicing physicians showed that of 273 cases of aplastic anemia that occurred in connection with this antibiotic, 118 occurred when this was the only drug taken. On the other hand, among 51 cases of aplastic anemia that were observed in patients taking tetracycline, only one occurred in patients receiving that antibiotic alone.[33] Since chloramphenicol and tetracycline are both broad-spectrum antibiotics and tend to be given for the same types of illness, these findings dispose of the argument that the blood dyscrasias accompanying the administration of chloramphenicol occur as a result of an infection that was present before chloramphenicol was given. The one case reported in association with tetracycline was probably an instance of idiopathic aplastic anemia (aplastic anemia of unknown cause), sometimes observed in patients who have not been taking any drugs.

The Registry of Adverse Reactions was also valuable because it put in the hands of the Council on Drugs up-to-the-minute statistics that it could use to keep before the medical profession the dangers inherent in giving certain drugs and the kinds of adverse reactions that would be likely to occur.

Finally, the adverse reactions program of the Council on Drugs was an important step toward more exact reporting. It led to systems such as those later initiated in several hospitals, where special personnel are assigned to ferret out every adverse reaction and computer methods are used to tabulate every dose of every drug administered to every patient under observation. Because these projects are expensive, they cannot be easily undertaken by the AMA; those that are in operation are being financed by either the Public Health Service or the FDA.

But the reporting of adverse reactions is not an end in itself; its purpose is to get doctors to prescribe certain drugs less often, to monitor them more carefully, and to treat the reaction more efficiently when it appears. The articles published under the auspices of the Council on Drugs have been helpful in this respect, but they are not enough. Persuasion or enforcement may sometimes be necessary, and this can best come from the doctor's peers. For this reason, the Council on Drugs requested the Joint Commission on the Accreditation of Hospitals to recommend that every hospital set up a mechanism for reporting adverse reactions to drugs, which the commission did in December 1964. Most hospitals have appointed committees for this purpose, and they will be discussed further in Chapter 13.

When the Seal of Acceptance program was in effect, the name of the drug was negotiated between the Council on Pharmacy and Chemistry and the manufacturer and became the one that was used in *NNR* and in all advertisements in AMA journals. Also, it was almost always adopted when the drug was eventually placed in the *USP*. This gave the council bargaining power that it lost when it no longer awarded the Seal of Approval. To regain bargaining power, the council and the *USP* in 1961 formed a joint Committee on Nomenclature. In 1964 this was broadened to include a representative of the *NF* (*The National Formulary*) and the name changed to the United States Adopted Names Council. The AMA continued to provide the expert staff for this operation. Since the Drug Amendments Act of 1962 gave the Secretary of Health, Education and Welfare the power to choose a nonproprietary (generic) name for a drug if he did not consider the one in use to be suitable, this council was enlarged again in 1967 to include a representative of the FDA. The present agreement is that the Commissioner of Food and Drugs will accept any name adopted unanimously. If there is disagreement, he reserves the right to designate an official name.[34]

Thus we see the gradual evolution of a regulatory process begun by a private group and strengthened by joining hands with other groups and eventually with government. The private groups, representing as they do the physicians, the pharmacists, and the drug industry, continue to have considerable influence on policy and the selection of individual names, and yet the requirements of government as they reflect the interests of the public are served without complete government controls. In another much larger arena, this happy liaison has not been achieved. I refer to the relationship of the AMA to the control by the federal government over the marketing of drugs.

No one could have fought harder for the first federal law that regulated drugs than the officers of the AMA and its Council on Pharmacy and Chemistry. In announcing the formation of the Council on Pharmacy and Chemistry in 1905, the Board of Trustees complained that the number of nostrums bewildered the physician and made it impossible for him to distinguish between them and ethical drugs. "In other countries," they reported, "either the government or an authoritative body, such as the French Academy of Medicine . . . controls such matters, but here nothing is done, and the result is that our profession is being humbugged. . . ."[35] When the exposures of the muckrakers and the idealism of the progressives aroused the country to the danger of dirty and decayed foods and of impure and dangerous drugs, their motives were hand in glove with the AMA's campaign for the abolition of quack remedies and secret formulas and for truth in advertising of drugs to physicians and the public. By publishing articles in its journal, by persuading doctors to write to their congressmen, and by lobbying directly, the AMA worked shoulder to shoulder with the reformers, the women's groups, the consumer groups, and with Dr. Harvey Wiley, the indefatigable head of the Bureau of Chemistry of the Department of Agriculture, which was to have jurisdiction over the regulation of drugs. When in 1906 the Pure Food and Drugs Act was finally passed, the editor of the AMA journal exulted: "The law is an evidence of the fact that our national legislature can not be bought."[36]

A few weeks later, however, he pointed out some of the deficiencies in the law and urged state laws to supplement the federal law; otherwise "Kopp's Baby's Friend can still carry on its mission of killing babies and making money for its owner in Pennsylvania, in other states the morphin [sic] it contains will make it unprofitable to push. . . ."[37]

Another indication of the AMA's attitude toward the federal government in those days was the statement of the Board of Trustees: "We have reason to believe that if the American Medical Association requests it, a semi-official recognition of this Council [the Council on Pharmacy and Chemistry] will be made by the government."[38] And it has already been noted that among the fifteen members of the first council, three were from the federal government.

When a decision of the Supreme Court in 1911 narrowed the interpretation of the labeling provisions of the act so as to make them almost worthless, the AMA immediately urged the President and the Congress to pass the necessary law, which they did in the form of the Sherley Amendment in 1912.

During the next few years relationships remained close. The AMA and the Bureau of Chemistry of the Department of Agriculture advanced toward their common goal by a series of lateral passes. They kept each other informed of proposed or desired legislation and lobbied for it side by side; Wiley spoke and Simmons editorialized against the same quack remedies; the Department of Agriculture analyzed dubious drugs for the AMA, and the AMA rounded up consultants for the Bureau of Chemistry.[39]

In 1928, when the FDA was attacked for allegedly co-operating unduly with manufacturers by allowing the sale of what was called "impure" ergot, the AMA vigorously defended the FDA. That agency, with the help of the majority of the medical profession, was able to show that it had acted correctly and as strictly as it could within the limitations of the law.[40]

It was becoming increasingly obvious, however, that the rules of the game were favoring those who wanted to skirt the law. In 1933, when Senator Copeland introduced a bill for stricter regulations, *The Journal of the American Medical Association* declared: "The medical profession should support this legislation with all the strength that it possesses."[41] It failed to pass. When Senator Copeland introduced another bill in 1935, the AMA Board of Trustees recommended that such a law should provide for registration of drug companies with government regulation of "all forms of drug advertising."[42] Subsequent bills were supported by the AMA even though the journal complained that one of the bills had been subjected to "plastic surgery in the legislative operating rooms" until it had become "an asthenic, chinless and impotent monstrosity."[43] In 1938, after the Elixir of Sulfanilamide tragedy (described in Chapter 10), a bill was finally passed. Even then the AMA complained that the bill was not strong enough because the Department of Agriculture was given no control over the advertising of drugs to physicians.[44]

After the passage of the 1938 Food, Drug and Cosmetic Act, the Council on Pharmacy and Chemistry continued to co-operate with the Department of Agriculture's successor as a regulator of food and drugs, the FDA. It described itself as an "organization qualified to express and crystallize the voice of medical experts concerning the standards, actions, indications and danger of drugs" and stated that its fact-finding and educational functions complemented the enforcement function of the FDA.[45] Other signs of partnership were the recruiting of two secretaries of the council from the staff of the FDA, the collaboration of the two staffs on an article explaining how drugs should be tested,[46] and the continued presence of representatives from the government on the Council on Pharmacy and Chemistry.

As late as 1953 the AMA apparently approved of stronger regulation by the FDA because it originated a bill, which eventually became law, authorizing the FDA to inspect pharmaceutical laboratories without first obtaining the permission of the proprietors.[47]

Yet six years later it had done an about-face. For when

Senator Kefauver began his hearings on the prices of drugs and the practices of the drug industry, the AMA was lined up solidly with that industry and against changes in the laws. The provision that the drug manufacturer had to prove his claims of efficacy before he could market a drug drew fire from the AMA because ". . . a drug's efficacy varies from patient to patient. . . . [H]ence any judgment concerning this factor can only be made by the individual physician who is using the drug to treat an individual patient."[48] This was patently at variance with a statement approved by the Board of Trustees in a report to the House of Delegates in 1954, which said: "The average physician has neither the time nor the facilities to experiment with new drugs in order to determine their proper indications for use. . . ."[49]

The AMA also opposed the portion of the proposed law requiring that the Secretary of Health, Education and Welfare determine whether the therapeutic effect of a modification of a drug for which a patent application had been made was significantly greater than that of the drug so modified.[50] This position, too, was contrary to the statement transmitted to the House of Delegates by the Board of Trustees in 1920, which complained that ". . . the profits to be made from the sale of a proprietary medicine on which the manufacturer holds a monopoly are usually large—sometimes enormous."[51] Nor was the AMA's new attitude toward patents consistent with its opposition in 1917 to granting the Bayer Company a renewal of the patent on aspirin. At that time the AMA had protested: ". . . practically no other country in the world . . . would grant a patent on either acetylsalicylic acid [i.e., aspirin], the product, or on the process for making that product. The United States granted both!"[52]

It is not my purpose to debate the merits of the American Medical Association's stand, but rather to try to understand the reason for this change of heart. It has been seen that drastic changes were made in the policies of the Council on Pharmacy and Chemistry around 1955, and now we see that a similar shift of opinion had taken place somewhere between 1938 and 1959 in the desire to collaborate with the federal government in regulating drugs. Why did the AMA abandon the Seal of Acceptance program?

One reason given by the critics of the AMA was the loss of income from advertising in AMA journals under the program. In 1953 a marketing opinion firm, Ben Gaffin and Associates, after surveying attitudes toward the AMA journals, reported to the AMA: "The advertisers, in general, feel that the AMA, especially through the Councils, distrusts them and views them as potential crooks who would become actively unethical if not constantly watched."[53] The Gaffin firm contended that advertising was important to the AMA, since advertisers had paid over 3 million dollars into its coffers in 1952, and yet since 1948 advertising space had increased 40 per cent in the "throwaway" journals (those that are sent to the physician free of charge) and only 3 per cent in the AMA journals. Since the former placed few or no restrictions on the content of advertising, the Gaffin firm recommended that the councils that awarded the Seal of Acceptance should speed up their evaluations of drugs, foods, and devices, should sell the physician on prescribing products that carried the Seal of Acceptance, and should loosen their restrictions on the advertising of mixtures and the use of trade names in advertising in AMA publications. Mr. Gaffin later claimed that his survey led to the "eventual dropping of the 58 year old council Seal of Acceptance program," and Senator Kefauver pointed to the rapid rise in the AMA's advertising revenues after the abandonment of the seal program, from $4,184,000 in 1955 to $7,997,000 in 1960.[54]

But the AMA witnesses vigorously denied that the survey had anything to do with the dropping of the seal program, and pointed out that the rise in advertising income began in 1953.[55] A study of the sources of AMA income from 1949 to 1960 shows advertising revenue remaining constant from 1949 to 1952, rising slowly from 1952 to 1955, then shooting up rapidly until 1959. The rapid rise was at least partly the result of the change in advertising policies, yet at the same time the methods of selling advertising were improved and the format of the journal was dressed up. Also, advertising in nonmedical magazines rose during the same period.[56]

In their turn, AMA witnesses gave several reasons why the seal program was dropped. They claimed that it took so much time that the Council on Pharmacy and Chemistry could not keep up with new drugs and that some manufacturers were unwilling to submit new drugs for consideration because acceptance took so long and because doctors used their drugs without a Seal of Acceptance.[57] Instead Dr. Ernest Howard said, the council was told: "Gentlemen, expand your horizon; look at drugs as a whole. Your objective is to study drugs and give your honest, valid, authentic opinions to the medical profession as effectively, as readably, as quickly as possible."[58]

Two other reasons given by Dr. Howard for the abandonment of the seal program were: ". . . it was too arbitrary, and too much authority was vested in one body," and, finally, he mentioned that there were certain legal problems.[59] By this it is presumed that he meant the likelihood of suits, since, as has been seen, the AMA had been subject to suits and threats of suits ever since it began evaluating drugs.

What can we make of these accusations and counteraccusations? It should be noted first of all that Ben Gaffin and Associates did not suggest dropping the seal program. They took a hard look at it, however, and apparently when the Board of Trustees also looked they decided that the game wasn't worth the candle. Whether they anticipated any rise in advertising revenue if they dropped the program we shall never know, but the possibility may have entered their minds. There is no evidence, however, that the pharmaceutical industry maneuvered the AMA out of the seal program. Morris Fishbein wrote at the time that some of the leaders of that industry "are convinced that such a decision would bring about chaos in the industry."[60]

Yet once the change was made, the AMA used it as a selling point. Dr. George Lull, the secretary and general manager, told the Pharmaceutical Manufacturers Association in 1957: "The consideration of advertising has been taken out of the jurisdiction of the council [on drugs]. . . . The former official rules of the council have been superseded entirely. . . ."[61] At present the staff members who decide on the admission of advertisements to the AMA journals are guided by the council's evaluation of drugs, but they no longer consult with members of the council. While I was a member of the council for seven years and chairman for three years, I was never asked for my opinion regarding a single advertisement. One physician on the staff of the Department of Drugs is at present assigned to the advertising staff as a consultant, but all decisions are in the hands of persons who are paid by the AMA and whose ultimate responsibility is to the administrators of the AMA.

Dr. Howard asserted that the dropping of the seal program challenged the councils to expand their horizons. It is true that the emphasis upon evaluating the drugs that were submitted by manufacturers for approval tended to shunt aside other drugs which might need equal or greater attention. Yet this did not have to be. Sometimes when a poor drug had been blatantly advertised to physicians, the council would evaluate it and publish its findings in the absence of a request, or of any co-operation, from the manufacturer. For instance in 1937, "prompted by the receipt of numerous inquiries," the Council on Pharmacy and Chemistry examined a drug called Larodon, even though the manufacturer did not submit the drug for consideration. It asked a consultant to review the literature; he was "unable to find any article concerning the chemical or experimental examination of Larodon. . . ." Consequently the council declared the drug unacceptable for *NNR* and stated that if the firm had "evidence to support the claims made, it should make this available to an impartial body such as the council before launching such a vigorous campaign of advertising to the medical profession."[62]

The council had resolutely refused to evaluate mixtures. Perhaps this was a blind spot, but it could have been cured without dropping the seal program.

The claim that the seal program vested too much authority in a small group is one that will always be made by the regulated against the regulators. The mission of the council demanded tough-minded men. It also demanded experts in the area of therapeutics, which the administrators of the AMA were not. If the AMA was to function as a professional body, it had to depend upon its unique ability to bring in experts who would work without compensation for the public good. One important recompense for such voluntary efforts was the knowledge that what they did counted for something. They could hardly make their opinions count if they couldn't affect the drug companies' actions. In the last analysis the Board of Trustees had the power it needed if it considered the council's actions too arbitrary; it had the power of appointment.

The legal problems that Dr. Howard spoke about were presumably suits or threats of suits against the AMA. When we consider the barrage of suits that had been thrown against it in the early years of the council's existence and from which the AMA had emerged vindicated, honored, and applauded for its pains, it seems absurd that threats of more suits should stop it when it had proved its worth to the profession, to the industry, and to the public for half a century, unless the original drive had been blunted and the original dedication turned aside.

Perhaps there was also a fear that, having been successfully sued by the federal government on the charge of conspiracy in restraint of trade in relation to medical care, the AMA might be sued on the same basis in relation to the limitation of advertising within its journals. This is an ever-present risk in any program of regulation by a nongovernmental agency, but certain safeguards may be taken against it. The public interest must always be clearly in the forefront of such a program, and the regulation must be fair, impartial, and based on accepted criteria. Although it seems obvious that these criteria had been met in the Seal of Acceptance program, it is possible that the trustees of the AMA, skittish and on the defensive after what they considered one unjust attack, did not want to lay themselves open to another. Whether the federal government would have challenged their Seal of Acceptance program is debatable. The American Dental Association, as we shall see later, has a similar program that is still active.

Can we find any more likely reasons why the Seal of Acceptance program was abandoned? Let us see. The Council on Pharmacy and Chemistry was started because doctors were bewildered with the array of drugs presented to them, often without identification beyond a trade name, composed of mixtures containing worthless ingredients, frequently harmful to the patient, and sometimes downright dangerous. The doctors themselves had at that time little training in pharmacology and some had no experience in treating patients when they left medical school. During the ensuing fifty years the picture changed, owing in part to the work of the councils of the AMA; physicians were better educated, the drug industry became more scientifically based and more responsible, and the federal food and drug acts of 1906 and 1938 required that drugs be identified, that they be manufactured according to certain standards, and that they be shown to be safe before they could be sold. These changes had been opposed, but it is significant that of the ten rules adopted by the Council on Pharmacy and Chemistry in 1905, all of them were routinely obeyed by 1955 except Rule 6, which stated that "no article will be admitted or retained about whose therapeutical value the manufacturer or his agents make unwarranted, exaggerated or misleading statements."[63] Even here, the companies had become so sophisticated in writing labels and advertisements, and used such ambiguous language, that a statement that seemed false or misleading to one physician seemed reasonable to another.

But after World War II the pharmaceutical industry in America had grown to giant size, and hundreds of new synthetic drugs flooded the market. With this came the Madison Avenue techniques of salesmanship, the ambiguous phrase, the sly suggestion, the half-truth, the insinuation that the drug advertised was the best and safest the doctor could use. The burden of time and money on the council and its staff became heavier and heavier; likewise the burden on the AMA's Chemical Laboratory. This had been originally set up to determine the identity of secret remedies. Under the AMA's vigorous attack these had diminished almost to the vanishing point, but the laboratory was now swamped with testing the purity of new drugs that were pouring out of the factories and a multitude of older products made by small firms who sold them under generic names and wanted the prestige that came from displaying the Seal of Acceptance. Did the Seal of Acceptance beside the name of a drug guarantee that every batch was pure? If so, the AMA could not possibly do the job.

Thus by 1955 it had become clear that the task facing the council was too big. A change of direction was needed, new objectives, new methods, new horizons, in fact, and perhaps new dedication.

But was the dedication there? There were some hints that the council was losing its steam. It had stopped publishing three books, several editions of which had been popular with practicing physicians: *Useful Drugs, The Epitome of the U.S.P. and National Formulary,* and *Glandular Physiology and Therapy.* It had stopped requiring that a drug could be advertised in AMA journals by its generic name only, and it had been unable to persuade the Board of Trustees to continue giving *NNR* to medical students. It had not pushed the grants program for therapeutic research, so that this was taken from the council and finally discontinued altogether. Perhaps, also, it had depended too much for its drive upon its chairman, Dr. Torald Sollmann, who had been on the council since its formation and who, though still remarkably vigorous, could not be expected to sprint at top pace forever.

For a private agency to be successful in a regulatory venture, five forces are necessary: consecration, crusading, consistent pressure, clubs, and cash. One needs only to read the editorials in the AMA journal in the early decades of the century to be convinced that the consecration was there. And to follow the speeches and the actions of Simmons and Fishbein, to watch how they braved criticism, vilification, and legal prosecution is to see militant, courageous crusaders in action. But Simmons died, Fishbein was dropped from the AMA staff and wasn't replaced by an equally militant champion, and eventually all staff members of the AMA were removed from the council.

The third force, continuous pressure, was applied in the

early years of the council when a chairman, such as Torald Sollmann, remained at the helm for many years and when the editor of the journal attended every meeting, but this force was effectively braked when the term of membership in councils was limited and chairmen could serve for only three years.

Regulation seldom if ever succeeds by persuasion alone; some kind of club is needed. In the case of drugs the Seal of Acceptance was that club. It had helped to keep the big companies in line, while the smaller companies scrambled to be in the ranks with them. The club was not big enough, but it could have been made larger. The club was there if the AMA wanted to swing it.

Finally, a program of regulation takes cash and lots of it, and the lack of cash may be the real rock on which the seal program foundered. In 1955 the AMA had just come through the searing experience of being prosecuted for a criminal violation of the antitrust laws, and had been convicted. The fine it had to pay was trivial, but the costs of the legal battle had not been. Moreover, the AMA was mounting a costly campaign to prevent government payment for medical care. And the accusation by the government that the AMA was restraining trade might well be echoed by some drug company whose products were not approved by the AMA, and this would cost more money! Added to this was the glimpse of that hoard of gold representing potential advertising from which the AMA was barred by the seal program. What could be simpler than to cut the Gordian knot, abolish the seal program, and with one bold stroke cure all these financial ills?

Whatever the real reasons for the abandonment of the seal program, it is apparent that the zeal that had in the past generated consecration, crusading, and consistent pressure was gone, that the cash drawer was low and might get lower. And so the club was thrown away.

What of the future? We have seen that the council began to move forward in the educational period after a preliminary interval of tacking back and forth. It improved its communications to practicing physicians, pioneered a program of reporting adverse reactions, and continued to bite into the problem of obtaining simple names for drugs by borrowing teeth from the *USP* and *NF* when it joined them to form the United States Adopted Names Council. Yet these steps have not been enough. When one questions practicing physicians in various sections of the country, as I have done, most of them have only vague notions of what the council is doing, many confess that they do not read the council columns on drugs and do not buy *New Drugs*. And they usually look elsewhere for their information on adverse reactions. Either the informational program to the practicing physician must be improved or else beaming information to him is not enough. Where, then, should the AMA set its sights for the future?

The Council on Drugs has directed its course since 1955 toward informing the physician about drugs. To this end it changed its publication *New and Nonofficial Drugs* to *New Drugs* and included more information of interest to the practicing physician. It is at present working on a book called *AMA Drug Evaluations* (*ADE*), in which it expects to give the practicing physician information about all of the drugs that are available on the market and to compare the efficacy and safety of drugs, indexing them by generic and brand names.[64] Such a book is badly needed, and if well written and kept up to date it could become the *vade mecum* of the practicing physician.

In this book, for the first time, the Council on Drugs is evaluating a number of mixtures of drugs. Some mixtures are valuable for therapeutic reasons, but most are prescribed because it is convenient for the patient to take fewer medications or because it is easier for the doctor to prescribe by a single name. It follows, then, that some of these mixtures are justified, but not all. Whether this figure should be 5 per cent or 75 per cent (and I believe it is closer to the former), physicians will continue to prescribe mixtures, as they do now, on the basis of advertising until some authoritative body evaluates them and gives the practicing doctor the information. Now that many of its former activities are being taken care of by the FDA, the

Council on Drugs is in a position to do this. And as a respected, impartial body it will be listened to.

In connection with *ADE* the council should publish information on the prices of drugs. This can be done in the volume itself and can be kept up to date by supplements. Without question, a book as valuable as this in other respects cannot afford to ignore the importance of the cost of drugs to the patient. Since differences in the physiologic availability of various preparations of the same drug have been recognized, it is important that *ADE* also include this information where data are available, and indicate those drugs for which differences in absorption are not significant.

The volume of advertising in AMA journals has not been adversely affected by recent federal laws and regulations. In the first three months of 1961, *The Journal of the American Medical Association* contained 1,431 pages of advertising, of which 1,151 were purchased by companies manufacturing drugs.[65] A count of the pages for the same period in 1968 yielded 1,438 and 1,172 pages, respectively.

But the AMA's functions have changed since the FDA is monitoring all advertisements to see that they provide full disclosure of the adverse effects of a drug and that they conform to the statements in the approved labeling. The AMA may go farther and insist that the advertisements in its journals be more factual, more accurate, and more complete than the FDA does, but in most cases this will mean wasted energy. It could judge in matters of taste, however, and eliminate the nude and the bizarre where they are irrelevant and in poor taste. It might stimulate advertisements that are more informative and thus more welcome to the doctor by making awards to advertisers for the advertisements that are most helpful in improving the doctor's treatment of patients.

The missions of a quasi-official agency—one that performs a public function even though it is not directly responsible to an official governing body—are *pioneering*, experimenting with new methods, demonstrating their effectiveness, and then turning them over to governmental units to carry out on a larger scale; *co-operating*, collaborating with governmental agencies; and *supporting*, stimulating, encouraging, championing, and, if necessary, criticizing public agencies so that they perform in the public interest. The AMA, acting mainly through its Council on Drugs, has succeeded in some of these objectives and failed in others.

As a pioneer, the AMA Council on Pharmacy and Chemistry initiated the process of evaluating drugs and accepting those it considered worthwhile. The council's identification of secret formulas and the clinical monitoring of drugs that its program necessitated paved the way for the Food and Drug Act of 1938, which required that the safety of a drug be proved before it could be marketed.

Dropping the Seal of Acceptance program probably increased the need for the Kefauver-Harris amendments. Had the council's program under the Seal of Acceptance been strengthened instead of dropped, it is likely that when the federal government tightened its laws, it might have included a working arrangement with the AMA, much as it had accepted the standards set in the *USP* and the *NF*.

The program of monitoring adverse reactions to drugs initiated by the Council on Drugs pointed up both the advantages and defects of voluntary reporting and pioneered the more extensive programs that are being initiated by the FDA.

Regarding the second mission, collaboration between the Council on Drugs and the FDA and their predecessors was at one time open, friendly, free, and productive. The olive branches have withered of late, although in one area, the naming of drugs, the programs of the two groups have dovetailed completely.

In its supportive mission, the AMA has pushed in different directions at different times. It encouraged and supported the federal government in the regulation of drugs up to the 1950's. Since then, it has opposed as often as it has supported, and criticized more often than it has praised.

The abandonment of the Seal of Acceptance program was followed by an avalanche of advertising revenue for the AMA. In 1968 its total income was over 30 million dollars, and of this, nearly 12 million dollars, or approximately 40 per cent, came from advertising.[66] Whether as a result of this, or because the scarcity of physicians and general prosperity has kept doctors' incomes at a high level for several decades, the AMA has moved far to the right politically since the 1920's.[67]

According to James G. Burrow the shift in political philosophy began when the AMA changed its attitude toward compulsory health insurance from exploratory interest to violent hostility between 1917 and 1920.[68] The battle was fought in the press, in the hustings, and in the halls of Congress for several decades after this, spotlighted by the prosecution of the AMA under the antitrust laws in 1938 and reaching its high water mark recently with the passage of Medicare.[69] It was only human, therefore, that while the AMA and one branch of the federal government were locked in a violent struggle, in which the AMA believed it was fighting for the survival of American medicine, the AMA would suspect the motives of other branches of the government, as shown by the interest of the Public Health Service in increased medical manpower, the strong financial support of the nation's medical schools by the National Institutes of Health, and the increased push toward stricter regulation of drugs by the FDA. To turn the other cheek toward the FDA after being slapped by the federal government was more than the doctors could do; the best their spokesmen could manage was to present a polite but frosty mien when it was necessary to meet on professional matters.

The achievements as well as the shortcomings of the past can point the way for the AMA in the future. Let us see what it can do now to further each of its functions: pioneering, co-operating, and supporting.

Much pioneering remains to be done. The problems of collecting data on drugs are by no means solved by the present emphasis upon the computerizing and instant transmission of data to any place in the country. The weak link is getting the facts in the first place. The FDA is supporting systems of reporting adverse reactions in certain hospitals, and the Public Health Service is supporting others; but these represent only a small fraction of all the patients treated, and they also involve special groups of patients. The AMA could experiment with a program in a few smaller hospitals or in the offices of some general practitioners, for instance. It could encourage a system of collaborative reporting by the physicians and pharmacists in a small town. The possibilities are endless.

If we know very little about the reporting of adverse reactions, we know even less about the way physicians use drugs and why. The AMA could encourage and sponsor studies of drug usage in hospitals and in doctors' offices, and the factors that influence doctors to change their habits.

The question of who is qualified to be an investigator of drugs in the early phases has not been settled. Nor is the FDA in a position to tackle it except by detecting investigators who are grossly careless or patently dishonest. The Council on Drugs together with the Council on Medical Education might study the present-day testing of drugs and from those studies formulate guidelines for the training and qualifications of physicians who should make the preliminary tests of drugs in the future.

Opportunities for co-operation are also waiting to be grasped. The Council on Drugs might establish panels of experts who would be available to give the FDA their opinion on a particular problem on short notice. I see no reason why members of the staff of the FDA and the Division of Biological Standards of the Public Health Service should not be members of the Council on Drugs as they were in the past, and members of the staff of the Department of Drugs of the AMA might well be members of the Advisory Council of the FDA. It is time to return to the era of mutual trust and helpfulness that was formerly so productive.

Much remains to be done in adopting simple, pronounceable, and recallable generic names for drugs. The AMA through the United States Adopted Names Council could insist on shorter names and back up its demands by polling practicing physicians to find out how well they work on the firing line. It should consult with experts in speech so as to avoid combinations of sounds that make pronunciation difficult. It should find a way, by seeking a special law if necessary, to pre-empt certain words and syllables for official use. Finally, it should tackle boldly the problem of simple names for mixtures of drugs. No doctor is going to write "norethynodrel with mestranol" for a contraceptive when he can write "Enovid."

The evaluation of a drug by the FDA is not complete. The FDA is not usually concerned with the relative efficacy of drugs nor how they work. These are fertile fields for the AMA, and it has already started to cultivate them more intensively by publishing *ADE*. Whether this will satisfy the FDA's requirement for a compendium that may replace the mandatory package inserts remains to be seen. (See Chapter 11.)

The Council on Drugs should evaluate drugs and compare them as it has done in the past, and it should boldly and unequivocally state its opinion. It should do this in spite of protests that "regulation of the pharmaceutical industry by pressure groups or self-appointed experts, even medical societies, is just as undesirable as would be such control of the practice of medicine."[70] Regulation, insofar as it is possible by the dissemination of information, should be welcomed by every responsible business or profession.

Finally, the AMA should augment its supportive function. Facts force the neutral observer to conclude that the AMA has swung around 180 degrees from being the champion of the consumer of drugs to being the champion of the drug industry. Undoubtedly the drug industry's interests do need defending; no governmental power, no matter how well intentioned, can be allowed to move unchecked. But a multi-million-dollar industry with intelligent and aggressive leaders is surely capable of defending itself. On the other hand, the consumers have few champions, and these are sometimes better intentioned than informed. Who can look out better for the consumer's interest in the area of drugs than the physician who is knowledgeable about drugs as a result of his training, who knows about consumers— his patients—from his daily work, and whose entire life is given over to caring for their interests? One of the great physicians of the nineteenth century, Rudolph Virchow, said that the physician is the natural advocate of the poor. Surely, he is the natural advocate for all consumers of drugs, rich or poor.

For these reasons the AMA should support those laws and

regulations that make for safe drugs and for more exact information about them reaching physicians and the public; it should help the public agencies as they try to make the laws and regulations work; it should criticize the government when it loses its zeal or flags in its efforts; and it should stand shoulder to shoulder with the government to hold back those who would shrug off the patient's discomfort or death for the sake of gold to line their pockets.

Drugs are a smaller part of the dentist's armamentarium than of the doctor's. Perhaps this explains why the dentists were latecomers in the field of regulation, although once they started they worked vigorously and skillfully. In 1927 the American Dental Association established a laboratory to standardize the composition of dental drugs and to check on secret remedies and inferior drugs. In 1930 it appointed a Council on Dental Therapeutics, which four years later published the first volume of *Accepted Dental Remedies*. Although this council stated that it was following the plan used by the Council on Pharmacy and Chemistry of the AMA, it departed from its model significantly in one respect: the dental council included "official" remedies from the USP and the NF and added to these the important drugs that had appeared since the last issues of those compendia.[71] Thus the dentist had a more complete list of drugs available to him in a single volume than the physician.

The Council on Dental Therapeutics also followed the AMA in adopting a Seal of Acceptance. But it is significant that the American Dental Association has not seen the necessity nor the advantage of dropping this seal; it is still awarded to accepted products and still required for advertising in the association's journal. Drugs are listed by their generic names; brand names are also given, but only those that are labeled and advertised in accordance with the council's provisions for acceptance.

The dental council has taken another step beyond the AMA's Council on Drugs; they have classified drugs according to their value to the dentist. Drugs are examined at the request of the

manufacturer or upon the initiative of the council. After evaluation they are placed in one of four categories:

GROUP A. Accepted products that will be listed in the book
and for which the Seal of Acceptance may be used
in advertising.

GROUP B. Products that lack sufficient evidence to justify inclusion in Group A for the present, but for which
there is reasonable evidence of usefulness and
safety.

GROUP C. Drugs for which the evidence is so limited or incon-
clusive that they cannot be adequately evaluated.

GROUP D. Unacceptable drugs.

Accepted Dental Remedies also contains chapters on general
therapeutic principles and sections explaining the relationship
of the important drugs in a particular class. Thus it serves as a
therapeutic guide for the dentist and appears to be a model of
what an enterprising professional association can do to aid its
practitioners in the field of therapy.

Why has the American Dental Association not found it
necessary to drop its Seal of Acceptance? Upon inquiry I have
been told that no such plan has been considered. Some cynics
might say that this is because a smaller percentage of its revenue
comes from advertising than is the case with the AMA. In 1967
receipts from journal advertising were slightly over $883,000, only
about one eighth of the total income of the association.[72] Others
might point to the smaller field to be encompassed. Whatever
the reasons, the Council on Dental Therapeutics has not only
retained its regulatory club but has boldly dared to classify drugs
according to their relative efficacy. The AMA might well take a
look at the program of its neighbor, ten blocks away.

*Some have said that it is not the business of
private men to meddle with government—a bold
and dishonest saying, which is fit to come from
no mouth but that of a tyrant or a slave.
To say that private men have nothing to do
with government is to say that private men have
nothing to do with their own happiness or misery.*
—MARCUS CATO

*The anger and disaffection of the intellectual,
once aroused, are a sword against which neither
the purse of the rich nor the law of the
mighty can ultimately prevail.*
—C. W. DE KIEWET

10

History of
Federal Regulation
of Drugs and
Biological Products

The flood of new products of the technological revolution, the distance of the consumer from the site of manufacture, and the awakening political power of the consumer have all combined to pressure governments into the regulation of food and drugs. In England the pressure reached the "legislation level" sooner than in the United States, and in 1872 the British Parliament declared it unlawful to sell an impure drug as a pure one. A later act passed in 1875, was worded so as to be more easily enforced and became the standard in that country until 1928.[1]

In the United States, a catastrophe sparked the first federal regulation of drugs. The city of St. Louis had been employing a bacteriologist for several years to prepare diphtheria antitoxin, when in 1901 ten children died from tetanus, which was shown to have been the result of contaminated antitoxin. The Medical Society of the District of Columbia led a fight for regulatory legislation, and in 1902 Congress passed a Biologics Control Act to insure that serums and vaccines sold in the District of Columbia or moving in interstate commerce would meet proper standards of purity, potency, and efficacy.

Meanwhile a groundswell of protest against filthy, fake, and fraudulently represented foods was being felt in Washington. Since the complaints came mostly from agrarian states, the Department of Agriculture undertook to study them. In 1887 the Chemical Division of that department, headed by Dr. Harvey W. Wiley, began reporting the results of the analyses of foods carried out in its laboratory.[2] These reports, comprising the famous Bulletin 13, were issued periodically during the next six years. They showed, for instance, that what was sold as pepper was mostly cracker crumbs, corn, and charcoal; that lard was adulterated with cottonseed oil; that molasses contained chloride of tin and bleaching agents; that "coffee beans" might be cereals or acorns or might be made of flour and sawdust.

Dr. Wiley became a militant crusader for legislation against impure foods, joined by farmer organizations, consumer groups, and many leading magazines. Drugs received less attention; he did not open a laboratory to test drugs until 1903, after the AMA was already vigorously fighting against secret and worthless remedies. Even as late as 1905 Wiley admitted that his laboratory had only scratched the surface so far as drugs were concerned.[3] Wiley did co-operate with the Council on Pharmacy and Chemistry of the AMA in its crusading, both as a council member and by supplying information. He also added speeches on drugs to his already hard-pressed schedule, and he pushed for legislation to control the purity of drugs as well as foods.

The attempts to get a food and drug bill through the narrow, crooked, and sometimes completely blocked legislative channels were numerous and frustrating. Between January 1879 and June 1906, when the Pure Food and Drugs Act was finally passed, 190 bills were introduced into Congress for protection regarding food and drugs.[4] According to James Harvey Young, each of the major federal food and drug laws was preceded by changes in technology and by crusading, compromise, and catastrophe.[5] The technology of foods—improvements in agriculture, processing, and transportation to distant cities—had been changing parallel to the technology of producing drugs, which has been discussed in previous chapters. Crusading for pure foods gathered momentum slowly, sparked first by the farmers and a few officials in the prairie states who saw firsthand how spoiled, contaminated, and adulterated food was being sold to a blind public. Soon they were joined by Wiley and his colleagues in the Department of Agriculture, by reputable food processors, and by medical and public health associations. Eventually came the muckraking books and articles in magazines such as *Collier's* and the *Ladies' Home Journal*. Consumer groups and women's groups also joined the ranks.

Yet all these forces were not enough to overcome the combined strength of the dishonest food manufacturers. Alongside them were the patent medicine makers, who peddled soothing syrups containing opium or huckstered highballs under the name of Lydia Pinkham's Vegetable Compound (20.6 per cent alcohol) and Hostetter's Stomach Bitters (44.3 per cent alcohol), or who adulterated phenacetin (patented and therefore expensive) with acetanilide (not patented and therefore cheap, but also dangerous to the point of being lethal in the amounts used).

Added to these were the congressmen, particularly from the Southern states, who opposed federal regulation of food and drugs on Constitutional grounds, claiming that the federal government could just as well regulate people's theological views or cut their toenails. Then, too, there were those who objected to a particular provision for fear it would be enforced too strictly, and those who wanted their pet interests advanced in a bill and opposed any legislation that helped their competitors. The oleomargarine and butter interests were at loggerheads, as were the manufacturers of baking powder made from cream of tartar and those whose baking powder contained alum.

Compromise became necessary, and many compromises were made in the effort to get some bill passed, but only an explosion could break the log jam. It came in the form of a novel, *The Jungle*, by Upton Sinclair, which described in detail the filthy and diseased meat in the Chicago packing plants. To the public this was a catastrophe. Aroused and angered, President Theodore Roosevelt demanded that a meat inspection bill be enacted and that the House of Representatives pass the bill it had been dawdling with for months. And it was passed, with much stronger provisions than those in the Senate's version. In the Conference Committee most of the House provisions prevailed, and on June 30, 1906, the Pure Food and Drugs Act was signed by President Roosevelt.

The new law was launched upon a sea of troubles. A major storm center was Harvey Wiley himself—Wiley the crusader, who believed, now that an act was on the books, he could win the battles in the courtroom as he had won them on the lecture platform; Wiley the dogmatist, who was convinced that those who disagreed with him were tools of the food and drug interests; Wiley the zealot, whose years as a propagandist for reform suppressed the qualities of judgment and temperateness necessary for an administrator in a regulatory agency. After many brushes with the Secretary of Agriculture and with Presidents Roosevelt and Taft, he resigned in 1912. His mantle fell upon Dr. Carl L. Alsberg, a biochemist. Alsberg combined an emphasis on the scientific underpinnings of the Bureau of Chemistry with an interest in strong regulatory practice. He placed regulatory matters under Walter Campbell, a lawyer by profession and an administrator by temperament. With some of the internal squabbling laid to rest, the Bureau of Chemistry was better able to proceed against the violators of the new law.

By this time another obstacle had appeared. In proceeding against Dr. Johnson's Mild Combination Treatment for Cancer the Bureau of Chemistry had shown that the claims for efficacy were baseless and dishonest. To their dismay, the district court ruled that the misbranding provision of the act did not apply to therapeutic claims. The Secretary of Agriculture asked President Taft to support a bill to remedy this, which he did, and in August 1912 Congress passed the Sherley Amendment, which classified a product as misbranded if claims in the labeling of therapeutic or curative effects were false and fraudulent. While this helped some, it still left the government in the difficult position of trying to prove that the manufacturer deliberately intended to defraud.[6]

In 1927 the regulatory part of the Bureau of Chemistry became an independent unit, at first the Food, Drug and Insecticide Administration and then the Food and Drug Administration, under Campbell's direction. In the three decades between the passage of the first and second major acts, the regulation of food and drugs was characterized by less headline-hunting after 1912, when Wiley left, by meticulous investigation into alleged violations of the law, and by careful attention to the details of enforcement. The main emphasis was on food, because so much was obviously crying to be done to protect the public against impure, spoiled, and adulterated foods and also probably because the public at that time knew little about the dangers of patent medicines and the doctors had so few effective drugs to offer as substitutes.

More and more, however, as the years went by, the frustrations piled up. The 1906 law had defined a drug too narrowly and had not included therapeutic devices or cosmetics. It had not required that the ingredients of a drug be listed on the label except for a few, such as alcohol and narcotics, but merely stated that they had to be correct if listed. It had authorized the enforcement of standards only for drugs listed in the official compendia. Also, advertising was completely uncontrolled. The Sherley Amendment had required the government to prove fraudulent intent in order to convict anyone for false therapeutic claims. Most important of all, dangerous drugs could still be legally sold, because drugs did not have to be tested for safety before marketing and the government did not have the power to move swiftly when a drug was found to be too toxic for use.

Soon after Franklin Roosevelt took office, a new bill was written at the behest of Rexford Tugwell, Assistant Secretary of Agriculture, and Walter Campbell. It was backed by the President and introduced by Senator Copeland. But it failed to pass, and so did three subsequent bills.

As before, the four C's were present. *Changes* in technology had produced many new drugs. Since 1906, food processing had grown enormously; the value of the products marketed by the regulated industries was ten billion dollars a year.[7] *Crusades* there were aplenty, although the armies were different. This time they were mainly the consumer organizations. The muck-rakers were the authors of books like *100,000,000 Guinea Pigs*, rather than magazine writers and newspaper editors. The AMA played a very minor role.

Compromise was needed, also. The drug industry was more solidly united against the early drafts of the new bill than it had been prior to 1906. In the first few years after that act became effective, the FDA found lots of flagrant violations against which it could and did proceed. These generated little opposition and in fact often earned plaudits from the more responsible manufacturers. In the later years, however, the FDA went to work on the more subtle and questionable infringements of the law. These often involved the larger and more responsible companies, and needless to say, these firms did not always agree on the interpretations of the law nor the objectives of the FDA. Thus, they were in no mood for a stronger bill.

Senator Copeland's second draft of the bill was more moderate than the first, so much so that it drew the wrath of the more militant crusaders, but the drug manufacturers were still not satisfied. They sensed by now that a bill of some kind would eventually be enacted, and they worked to make it as weak as possible. The manufacturers of proprietary drugs objected especially to placing the regulation of the advertising of food, drugs, and cosmetics under the FDA. By way of compromise, the Wheeler-Lea Amendments to the Federal Trade Act kept the control of drug advertising under the Federal Trade Commission while widening its powers to include unfair practices that could injure consumers in addition to those that harmed competitors.

Still there might have been no new food and drug act had it not been for a *catastrophe*. Sulfanilamide, dissolved in a commercial solvent, diethylene glycol, without tests for toxicity on the solvent or the finished product, was placed on the market in several Southern states. Before its lethal onslaught could be checked, it killed over a hundred persons, many of them children.[8] The FDA agent who investigated the firm that made and sold Elixir of Sulfanilamide reported: "The most amazing thing about the company was the total lack of testing facilities. Apparently they just throw drugs together and if they don't explode they are placed on sale."[9] Yet the gaps in the law were such that the proprietor could claim that he had done nothing illegal.

Congress moved to close the gaps. The new law widened the powers of the FDA in several fields. It broadened the definition of drugs by including substances used in patients to diagnose disease and to alter body functions or structures as well as to treat disease. It included cosmetics and therapeutic devices. As a specific response to the Elixir of Sulfanilamide tragedy it required that before any new drug could be marketed, proof of its safety be demonstrated by all reasonably applicable methods to the satisfaction of the FDA. The principle of testing before general use was followed in another area; only those coal-tar dyes that the FDA listed as safe could be used in foods, drugs, and cosmetics, and the FDA was to certify individual batches as safe. In the future all the active ingredients of a drug mixture had to be listed on the label, and the quantity or proportion of an expanded list of potentially harmful ingredients had to be stated. Labeling had to contain adequate directions for use. Warnings had to be placed on the labels of drugs that were habit-forming or subject to misuse. A drug was considered misbranded if the labeling was false or misleading in any particular; proof of fraud was no longer required. Other provisions strengthened the regulation of foods. Finally, the government was empowered to obtain an injunction when it needed to move swiftly. Although a compromise and although containing weaknesses, as became evident when attempts were made to enforce it, the Food, Drug and Cosmetic Act of 1938 was a giant step forward in the field of drug regulation.

The commissioner who had shepherded the new law through Congress, Walter Campbell, spent another six years getting the expanded program under way. He was followed in 1944 by Paul B. Dunbar, a Ph.D. in chemistry. He was succeeded by Charles W. Crawford, also a chemist, in 1951, and he in turn, in 1954, by George P. Larrick, who had climbed the administrative ladder from the position of inspector in thirty-one years. Under these leaders the agency developed a philosophy of quietly but firmly carrying out the spirit of the 1938 act. Where possible, voluntary compliance was obtained from individual companies or representatives of the industry, but whenever necessary the FDA did not hesitate to use its regulation-making authority and the powers of seizure, prosecution, and injunction to enforce the mandates of Congress as it saw them. All of this was done with a minimum of fanfare, so that the public and the medical profession hardly knew such an agency existed, a policy that was later criticized because, it was asserted, it resulted in minimal appropriations and consequent deficiencies in staff and facilities.

In the quarter-century after the act went into effect, approximately fourteen thousand applications for new drugs for human and veterinary use were received.[10] The development of the expertise to test these drugs stimulated technological progress in the pharmaceutical industry as well as in the FDA.

Problems were encountered along the way. Some of these were fought out in the courts and some resulted in new laws. The food and drug laws were based on the commerce clause in the Constitution, but where did interstate commerce end? Because the courts disagreed, Congress in 1948 passed the Miller Amendment, which gave the FDA jurisdiction over drugs and foods that were adulterated or misbranded anywhere between their manufacture in one state and their eventual purchase by the consumer in another.[11] Much of the strength of the 1938 act depended on the authority of the FDA to declare misbranded any drug the labeling of which was misleading or did not reveal significant facts about the drug. Labeling was defined as written, printed, or graphic matter on the article or container, or accompanying it. In 1948 the Supreme Court ruled that such printed matter actually "accompanied" an article even when sent in a separate container and at a different time. This ruling prevented dishonest promoters from using the subterfuge of sending drugs and labeling separately.

Because individual batches of insulin might vary in strength and because even a slight variation could mean life or death to a patient, the FDA sought authority to certify batches of insulin according to the standards of strength, quality, and purity set up by the *USP* (*United States Pharmacopeia*). The law authorizing this was passed in 1941, just before the patent on insulin expired. Since the holder of the patent had previously controlled the licensing of this drug and had been responsible for its potency and purity, this law undoubtedly prevented chaos in the therapy of diabetes. Certification was extended in 1945 to penicillin and later to other antibiotics, but here the FDA set the standards.

In one area the FDA did not make out so well. The Supreme Court in 1952 refused to require inspection of a food processing plant when the proprietor did not give permission. Although in 1953 Congress passed a law to remedy this, the FDA interpreted statements made during the congressional debate to mean that much essential information could be withheld from inspectors.

All in all, the story of the years between the acts of 1938 and 1962 was that of dedicated public servants struggling with a small staff and only fragmentary support from outside groups to protect the public as well as they could against large, well-organized, and politically powerful industries. This was made clear in 1955 in the report to the Secretary of Health, Education and Welfare made by a Citizens' Advisory Committee on the FDA. It recommended increases in personnel, in-service training, greater publicity on the objectives and actions of the FDA, programs for the investigation of the adverse effects of drugs, and an increase in the research activities of the FDA. Some of the recommendations were followed, including some increase in staff, but in general inadequate funds and the pressure of routine duties prevented much being done.

Meanwhile, technological change in the drug industry was accelerating. Not only were more drugs being produced, but they were in general more effective than in the past. Sophisticated procedures had been developed by the universities and the pharmaceutical companies for studying drugs in animals and to a lesser extent in people. Strapped by a limited budget, isolated from much contact with universities, subordinate in funds and number of personnel to the industries it regulated, the FDA looked mainly to consolidating its gains and improving its position in areas in which it had already been given jurisdiction, and did not reach out for more. Benjamin Franklin described its plight when he said: ". . . Those who govern, having much business on their hands, do not generally like to take the trouble of considering and carrying into execution new projects. The best public measures are therefore seldom adopted from previous wisdom, but are forced by the occasion."[12] The occasion was the bombshell of the Kefauver committee hearings, which burst on a startled drug industry and public.

Since 1957 the Subcommittee on Antitrust and Monopoly of the Judiciary Committee of the Senate, chaired by Estes Kefauver, had been investigating the reasons for and the effect of administered prices in the steel, automobile, and bread industries. Complaints of the high prices of drugs prompted the subcommittee to open hearings on the drug industry in December 1959. The more it investigated, the more problems it uncovered.

They involved not only prices, but deficiencies in the testing of drugs, lack of knowledge about the actions and adverse effects of drugs, misleading advertising, and resulting confusion in the minds of the physicians who did the prescribing. Thus crusading for a new law came this time mainly from a congressional committee, with help from those members of the practicing medical profession and the academic community who had been raising their lonely voices against these evils, along with a few dissidents in the FDA and the drug industry and some consumer groups. Hearings of the Subcommittee on Antitrust and Monopoly occupied nine months, from December 1959 through September 1960 and, together with exhibits, took up 16,505 pages.[13]

In getting to the core of truth, Senator Kefauver and the public were continually astonished as layer after layer of facts was peeled off and each layer put under the microscope of public inquiry. An examination of the facts required a look at costs, which showed that gross profits sometimes amounted to as much as 78 per cent of the income from sales, much higher than the profits made by most companies in other industries.[14] This required scrutiny of the costs of production, which revealed that costs for sales promotion for twenty-two companies took up 24.8 per cent of the sales income, while research costs involved only 6.3 per cent. This in turn demanded an examination of the underlying layer of monopoly and oligopoly, and inquiry as to whether these practices were in the public interest. The industry claimed that it would be stifled if laws were passed that lowered prices, but a parade of witnesses testified that most of the drugs marketed were not worth-while advances and that much of the so-called research was wasted.

When the high costs of selling drugs incited an inquiry into the reasons therefor, it was found that the average physician was deluged with drug advertising at the rate of 10.5 pieces of mail per day, and that it cost nine to ten dollars for a detail man to make a call on a doctor, or roughly 1.5 million dollars to make a single call on each practicing doctor in the country.[15] A look at advertising under the microscope of the congressional committee also revealed that advertisements were often misleading; that they often failed to refer to the possible dangers attendant upon the administration of drugs; indeed, that the drugs advertised had often been inadequately tested, so that the promoter could not really tell the doctors what they would or would not do; and that the drug companies tried to confuse physicians by giving long, unpronounceable generic names to drugs, so that the physician would think their drug with a short, snappy trade name was different from all other drugs.

Naturally these revelations attracted headlines, which Senator Kefauver did not discourage and in fact probably aided by the timing of the testimony. The public was aroused. That he was soaked and his doctor was duped was the message, right or wrong, that reached the man on the street.

The drug industry was horrified; its pride was injured; its purse was threatened. It sprang to the defense. It tried to justify its profits on high risks, on its contributions to the nation's health, on its record in research, on its part in educating the physicians. It paraded its own witnesses—economists, physicians, laboratory scientists (including Nobel Prize winners). During the first round of hearings it made a poor showing, probably because of the haste in which its case had to be prepared, but after Senator Kefauver had introduced a bill and hearings were held on that (from July 1961 until February 1962)[16] the industry presented its case more effectively, winning a commendatory headline from *Science*: "The Drug Industry Finally Has Its Day and Does Quite Well."[17] The drug companies agreed that information should be more widely disseminated to physicians and that the FDA should be able to run substandard drugs off the market; they even said they would go along with the provision that the efficacy of drugs be passed on by the FDA before they were marketed. But with a loud and unanimous voice they stubbornly opposed the slightest change in the patent laws or compulsory licensing of patents. The testimony in this second set of hearings took a curious twist when the AMA turned out to be more conservative than the drug industry, opposing the evaluation of efficacy by the FDA and insisting that the dissemination of information about drugs was the prerogative of the medical profession.[18]

The Kefauver committee hearings polarized the lay press according to whether a newspaper or magazine was conservative or liberal, pro or anti big business, anti or pro big government. The first groups called the hearings an inquisition and termed the testimony of the hand-picked witnesses "wild, irresponsible, sometimes untrue."[19] Those at the opposite pole said that the corporate giants (including the large drug companies) ". . . in undercutting the free market also undermine free society. Their power through advertising has reduced a free press to a caricature of its great pretensions. The drug companies also drug the public mind. . . ."[20]

Many medical journals were violently anti-Kefauver. Whether this was because they were mostly subsidized by advertisements from drug companies or saw in this legislation the bogey-man of federal control over the practice of medicine is an open question. They tended to condemn the whole affair as nothing but politics. *The New England Journal of Medicine*, however, true to its reputation for looking beyond the narrow interests of the day, stated: "Most of the principles embodied in the bill seem well defined to serve the primary purpose of protecting the health of the public."[21]

The journal *Science*, with remarkable prescience, noted that the bill introduced by Senator Kefauver fell naturally into two parts. One group of provisions would require the FDA to evaluate the efficacy of a drug in addition to its safety before it was marketed, to license manufacturers of drugs, to approve official names for drugs, which would be printed in such a way as to compete favorably with the trade name for the eye of the reader, to test individual batches of all antibiotics (rather than only a few as already provided for by law), to approve all printed matter accompanying the drug and all advertising, and to tell physicians directly about drugs "having the potentiality of particularly serious, dangerous or harmful effects." *Science* contended that these provisions involved "widely supported, long-discussed reforms," that they would improve the quality of medical care but not necessarily lower drug prices, and that because their need was apparent to so many well-informed people, the burden of proof that they did not benefit the public was on the opponents of the bill.

The second group of proposals would have required proof of

the therapeutic efficacy of molecular modifications or combinations of existing drugs before a patent was issued. They would also have required compulsory licensing of drugs three years after the patent was issued (and the date of issue would be the date when the drug was approved for marketing by the FDA). These provisions would have lowered drug prices, but their effect on the quality of medical care would have been doubtful, possibly even harmful. With regard to these provisions *Science* predicted that Congress would say: "Let's look into this thing more carefully before rushing ahead."[22]

And—after a lot of pulling and hauling and behind-the-scenes shenanigans—this is the way it turned out. Following Senator Kefauver's crusading there was the customary process of compromise, but it was accompanied this time by more than the usual amount of confusion. To begin with, President Kennedy's office arranged for a different and weaker bill to be introduced in the House of Representatives rather than supporting Kefauver's version, which had been introduced into the House by Congressman Celler. Then officials from the Department of Health, Education and Welfare met with Senator Eastland and other members of the Senate Committee on the Judiciary, but not with Senator Kefauver, to revise the bill Kefauver had sponsored. Out of this conference emerged a watered-down version of Senator Kefauver's bill that provoked a violent speech by Kefauver on the Senate floor and led to a repudiation of the revised version by the administration.[23] It looked like a weak bill or, more probably, no bill at all. Then came the catastrophe!

Beginning in 1959, doctors in Germany and in England had noticed an alarming number of cases in which children were born with abnormalities of the arms, legs, ears, or other organs. The commonest defects were seal-like flippers in place of the usual bones of the arm, forearm, and hands—indeed, the condition was called phocomelia, meaning seal-extremities. No cause could be found until Dr. Lenz of Hamburg reported in November 1961 that he suspected that thalidomide, taken by pregnant women, had caused them to have deformed babies. This drug, widely used as a hypnotic, had been first marketed in 1959 in Germany and then in other countries.

In the United States, because it alone among the major countries of the world required prior proof of safety, the drug was never marketed. Dr. Frances Kelsey and her colleagues of the FDA did not believe that the tests of animal toxicity correctly mirrored the effects on humans because the drug seemed to work differently in animals and humans, and she had become disturbed over some cases of peripheral neuritis in patients who had received thalidomide. Although she and her superiors were strongly and persistently pressured to release the drug, they resisted and were rewarded for their efforts when the reports from Germany and England showed the relationship between thalidomide and phocomelia. Later the drug was shown to produce other congenital abnormalities, such as missing ears, saddle-noses, and abnormalities of the gastrointestinal tract and heart. American children had been saved, except for a few born to mothers who had obtained the drug from other countries or from "investigator"-physicians in the United States.

The Wm. S. Merrell Co., which had been licensed by the German producers to market thalidomide in the United States (and was already marketing it in Canada), had supplied it to 1,126 physicians in this country for clinical trials. It proved impossible to locate some of the samples or even to find out who had been given the drug.[24] The newspapers, television, and radio diligently reported the gruesome details. The headlines screamed, the public was aroused, the drug manufacturers ran scared, and the opponents of a tough bill jumped for cover. In introducing to the Senate the bill that was to become the law, Senator Eastland made the understatement of the year when he said: "The bill [i.e., the weakened version] was reported to the Senate on July 19, 1962. Thereafter, as a result of the tragic thalidomide episode, the committee undertook a further review of the Food, Drug, and Cosmetic Act. . . ."[25]

The result was a greatly strengthened bill similar to the original Kefauver bill. Before it was passed, however, one significant addition was made from the floor of the Senate.

Senator Javits introduced an amendment that persons receiving drugs that had not yet been approved by the FDA must be informed of that fact, and he later justified this by stating: "I am for experimentation. I feel deeply that some risks must be assumed in experimentation. But we must hold the balance between personal dignity and personal responsibility and the right of the individual to know how his life is being disposed of, at least with his consent, and the virtues of experimentation."[26]

After some modification, this amendment was passed. Senator Kefauver introduced an amendment that would permit the Secretary of Health, Education and Welfare to require adequate tests in animals before a new drug could be tested in humans. After this was approved, he submitted amendments designed to change the patent laws with respect to drugs (which had been in his original bill, but had been omitted from the bill reported to the Senate). These were defeated. Finally came the vote on the bill itself, and it passed 78 to 0. In the incandescent light of thalidomide, no one had dared vote against it! As Senator Douglas said afterward, the vote was "a commentary on how time and history frequently bear out the views of some people. . . ." He concluded that ". . . because of the many tragedies . . . from the use of the drug thalidomide . . . it has been proved that the Senator from Tennessee [Kefauver] was right all the time and that the scoffers, scorners, and bitter opponents were wrong. . . . Certainly the American people will eternally be grateful to him."[27] After some further skirmishing in the House of Representatives and in the Conference Committee of the two chambers, the bill (now known as Public Law 87-781, the Drug Amendments of 1962, or the Kefauver-Harris Amendments) was passed and on October 10, 1962, was signed by the President.

When the smoke of the battle had cleared away, the new law was found to contain many important provisions. For the first time it required that establishments where drugs were manufactured be registered and subject to periodic inspection of their factories and, for prescription drugs, of their records of manufacture and testing. Even more important was the requirement that a drug be approved by the FDA as effective as well as safe before it could be marketed. The government's approval procedure was strengthened by the provision that the sponsor furnish substantial evidence of effectiveness "consisting of adequate and well-controlled investigations, including clinical investigations, by experts qualified by scientific training and experience to evaluate the effectiveness of the drug involved, on the basis of which it could fairly and responsibly be concluded by such experts that the drug will have the effect it purports or is represented to have. . . ." in the labeling. Approval of older drugs could be withdrawn, after a hearing, if new information appeared which seriously questioned the safety or efficacy of a drug; if there were an imminent hazard to public health this could be done in advance of a hearing. In testing new drugs, the experts would be required to "inform any human beings to whom such drugs, or any controls used in connection therewith, are being administered, or their representatives, that such drugs are being used for investigational purposes . . ." and were required to ". . . obtain the consent of such human beings or their representatives, except where they deem it not feasible or, in their professional judgment, contrary to the best interests of such human beings."[28]

All antibiotics had to be certified before being marketed, with certain exemptions for individual antibiotics for which sufficient experience in manufacture had been gained. The government was given the authority to designate an official name for a drug "in the interest of usefulness and simplicity"[29] and required to publish lists of official names. Information to physicians was covered by provisions that the labeling and inserts that accompanied each package be made available to any doctor who requested them, that advertisements contain the established name printed in type at least half as prominent as that used for the brand name, and that a true statement of information be given with respect to safety, efficacy, and contraindications.

The period since the passage of the 1962 act has been characterized by rapid changes in the top officials of the FDA, moves by the FDA to implement the far-reaching provisions of the act, tough talk and aggressive actions to impress upon the drug industry that the FDA would enforce the new act vigorously, and a series of hearings by congressional committees.

Many critics believed that the FDA, under Commissioner Larrick, has been "soft on industry." The commissioner was criticized for ostensibly tailoring the demands of his agency to the wishes of the larger drug companies instead of taking a positive stand and making them conform. Senator Humphrey wrote that the FDA's "principal lack in past years was not manpower; it was will power. Unlike its crusading founder, Dr. Harvey W. Wiley, the agency got into the habit of 'playing it safe.' "[30] And on the floor of the Senate he objected to the "turtle-like pace" of the FDA.[31]

Even in *Drug Trade News*, an organ of the drug and cosmetic industry, a reporter wrote in 1959: "The Larrick regime can be characterized as one of sweetness and light, togetherness, loving one's neighbor (industry and Congress) as one's self. This doesn't set well with some old-timers who remember Walter Campbell's mailed fist."[32] An official report of the Secretary of Health, Education and Welfare in 1960 admitted: "There can be no doubt that in the 15 years which have elapsed since World War II the FDA has moved toward industry in many respects."[33]

In spite of criticisms leveled at him during hearings of congressional committees and in spite of ill health, Commissioner Larrick stuck to his post until he had put the machinery in operation to implement the new drug amendments. In June 1963, regulations were issued that included requirements for new drug applications and for good manufacturing practices. Regulations for labeling and advertising were delayed because of objections from the drug industry, but these became final in April 1964. Commissioner Larrick also appointed Dr. Joseph Sadusk as Director of the Bureau of Medicine.

Dr. Sadusk speeded up the appointment of an advisory board and advisory committees and the awarding of contracts for gathering information that the FDA needed. Unfortunately he ran afoul of Congressman Fountain's subcommittee when he objected to producing the names of patients who had suffered adverse reactions from drugs and the transcription of the conversations of a meeting of an advisory committee. He believed that yielding on the first point would violate the confidential relationships between doctor and patient, and that yielding on the second would mean that he could no longer get top scientists to serve on advisory committees. Although ethically he was on solid ground, legally the Congress had the right to demand the information,[34] and in the end Congressman Fountain's committee got it.

In spite of this regrettable controversy Dr. Sadusk should be credited with upgrading the status of the physicians of the FDA and flagging the attention of practicing and academic physicians to the objectives and problems of the Bureau of Medicine. When he resigned, the new commissioner of food and drugs, the first M.D.-commissioner in four decades, took up the flag and waved it before the public as well as the medical profession.

Commissioner Larrick retired in 1965 after forty-two years of devoted public service in the FDA and its predecessor agency. He was succeeded by Dr. James Goddard, a career administrator in the Public Health Service, who was young, vigorous, forthright, and disposed to speak directly on issues that others might consider too delicate to touch. He did not hesitate to seize drugs, not only because of impurities, as had been done in the past, but also because their sponsors were promoting them with advertising that he considered misleading. He moved vigorously in administrative matters, also. He gave district directors more authority, eased the manpower crisis in the Bureau of Medicine by persuading the Public Health Service to lend him ninety-five physicians, veterinarians, and pharmacists who were fulfilling selective service obligations there. Most important of all, he arranged for the National Research Council to make a study of the efficacy of approximately three thousand drugs that had been passed on for safety under the 1938 act and now had to be evaluated for efficacy under the provisions of the 1962 act. On the other side of the coin, a reporter for the *Wall Street Journal* accused him of acting at times from misinformation and in haste. "The bold public pronouncement came far more readily than the vigorous followthrough,"[35] he added.

After two and a half years in the office, Dr. Goddard resigned and was replaced on July 1, 1968, by Dr. Herbert L. Ley, Jr. Dr. Ley's background was in research and teaching, and his last position had been in the Harvard School of Public Health. *Drug Trade News* predicted a change in the attitude of the FDA, saying: "The two men are totally different in appearance and personality. With Dr. Ley in the saddle, the 'glamour boy' image of FDA will disappear, but this may be the best thing that could happen at FDA at this time. . . . A period of quiet, firm and fair administration may be just what the doctor ordered."[36]

Firm and fair administration is what Dr. Ley attempted, but quiet it was not to be. Frequent Congressional hearings consumed much of his time; the pharmaceutical industry continued to oppose actions taken by the FDA to implement the 1962 Act, and, most important, a new administration came into office. The new Secretary of Health, Education and Welfare decided to transfer out of the FDA Commissioner Ley, his Deputy, and the Associate Commissioner for Compliance. Instead, Dr. Ley resigned on December 11, 1969. His successor was Dr. Charles C. Edwards, who had been successively a practicing surgeon, a staff member of the AMA, and an official in a firm of management consultants.

Secretary Finch was quoted as saying that he had great respect for Dr. Ley's scientific abilities but that Dr. Ley "had failed to furnish the necessary aggressive leadership,"[37] but another view was that the Secretary, worried over his own political future because of the many controversies in which the FDA was embroiled, decided to eliminate those who could be implicated in the agency's failure to satisfy its clamorous but diverging critics.[38]

The appointment of career administrators over a period of forty years and of one academically oriented commissioner gave the FDA some protection against the shifting winds of politics. Now, apparently, these safeguards have been stripped away. Perhaps the consumer will gain by this, but if so he will have to be more vocal than he has been in the past.

Of equal significance to the FDA was the reorganization of the Department of Health, Education and Welfare in 1968, which inserted an echelon between the commissioner of Food and Drugs and the secretary of the department. The FDA was placed in the newly formed Consumer Protection and Environmental Health Service, the administrator of which reported directly to the Assistant Secretary for Health. Although Secretary Cohen denied that this meant a downgrading of the FDA,[39] it seems certain that this will happen. Protests against the new status of the FDA have come from all sides, and at the present writing (December 1969) there are signs that the agency may be restored to its former rank. This I believe to be highly desirable. The reader can judge for himself after considering the activities of the FDA in the next chapter. But first let us take up the control of biological products.

The words "biological products" or "biologics" usually mean serums and vaccines used for the prevention, treatment, or diagnosis of disease, although the meaning has gradually been widened to include products similar to serums and vaccines that are used in the management of allergic conditions, and also some products prepared from blood.

In contrast to the fluctuating history of drug control, the history of biologics control has shown a steady growth of the philosophy and facilities of regulation as technological change demanded. True, there have been catastrophes that have thrust the control of biologicals before the public's eyes, but these have usually called for the acquisition of more technological knowledge and laws requiring that this knowledge be applied.

The first law that established biologics control as a function of the federal government followed such a catastrophe, as mentioned on page 188. Administration of this law was assigned to the Hygienic Laboratory of the Public Health Service. Eventually, as the Hygienic Laboratory became the National Institute and then the National Institutes of Health, a separate laboratory was established for the control of biologics; this in turn expanded into the present Division of Biologics Standards. When the laboratory first began its work, only three biological products were licensed: diphtheria and tetanus antitoxins and smallpox vaccine. In contrast, the Division of Biologics Standards now licenses over 300 products made by about 220 manufacturers.[40] The total budget of the Division is about 8 million dollars a year.[41]

The measures used for regulation include setting of standards for biological products; furnishing samples of biologicals, for use as reference standards, to establishments engaged in manufacturing or testing biological products (see Chapter 8); inspection of the establishments preparing biological products; licensing of establishments and products; and testing of individual batches.

The setting of standards is one of the reasons why a large staff is needed. To set standards properly the staff must be ready for a new vaccine or serum *before* it is perfected: in other words, it must carry on its own research. Devotion to this concept led the staff of the Hygienic Laboratory to manufacture a rabies vaccine, as a result of which they found that the encephalitis that sometimes follows the injection of this vaccine was caused by allergy to the rabbit brain in which the virus was grown. Unsuccessful "takes" from smallpox vaccines led to the development by the regulatory group of the present successful method of inoculating the vaccine, the "multiple-puncture" method. Research on adverse reactions to diphtheria antitoxin was responsible in the first decade of the twentieth century for the development by Dr. Milton Rosenau, director of the Hygienic Laboratory, of the "first sound theory ever advanced" to explain hypersensitivity reactions. Later, scientists in this agency developed vaccines for Rocky Mountain spotted and typhus fevers[42] and in recent years the first experimental live virus vaccine against rubella.[43]

Inspections of plants are made at least once a year by members of the scientific staff of the division, and more often when necessary. At this time both facilities and production methods are inspected, and records dealing with production and testing are reviewed.

Since the 1962 Drug Amendments Act went into effect, a sponsor, before beginning clinical investigation of a new biologic, must file with the division an investigational New Drug Application, just as he would make an application to the FDA for some other drug. The information contained in this application, plus the ongoing research of the scientists in the division, which has already been mentioned, enables these scientists to set the standards for a new biological before it is marketed.

Once the drug has been approved for marketing, samples obtained during factory inspections or by purchase are tested at intervals. When deficiencies or mistakes are found, they are almost always corrected by mutual agreement with the sponsoring company. The director of the division has testified: "In general there have been few problems with the larger producing laboratories. . . . In most cases where defects have been encountered these have been due to technological problems and enforcement is most readily accomplished by a process of voluntary compliance."[44] He added that in recent years the division had found a few criminal violations of the regulations on the part of some of the smaller establishments, particularly those marketing blood for transfusion. A staff of nonscientist inspectors was formed to deal with such cases, and convictions were obtained in some. An extreme weapon, which the division rarely uses, is the revocation of a company's license to manufacture biologicals, which, of course, would put the firm out of business.

The Division of Biologics Standards has functioned smoothly as a regulatory body and with little fanfare. Whether this is because it deals with only one basic discipline, because it needs to monitor relatively few biologics compared to the many drugs under the surveillance of the FDA, or because the division is highly oriented toward research with a relatively large professional staff is difficult to determine. Probably all three play some part.

The division has not been without its moments in the public eye, however. The outstanding example of this was in relation to the regulation of killed poliomyelitis vaccine. After the wide-ranging trials of killed poliomyelitis vaccine conducted under the auspices of the National Foundation for Infantile Paralysis were strikingly successful in showing the efficacy and apparent safety of the vaccine, production was begun by several commercial companies. Among these were the Cutter Laboratories. During a ten-day period in April 1955 approximately 400,000 persons were inoculated with the vaccine made by this company; in the next two months 94 cases of poliomyelitis occurred among the persons vaccinated and at least 166 among family and other contacts of the vaccinees. The Public Health Service, of which the Division of Biologics Standards was a part, immediately mobilized to meet the crisis. Cutter Laboratories was asked to recall all of its vaccine. Epidemiologic and laboratory studies led to the conclusion that certain lots of Cutter vaccine contained live virulent poliomyelitis virus. This was not the first experience that the Public Health Service had had with infectious poliomyelitis vaccine. In 1935 approximately 20,000 persons were given one or two vaccines developed independently by Drs. Kolmer and Brodie. Some persons who received each of the vaccines contracted cases of poliomyelitis that were traced to the vaccine.[45]

In all three instances the Public Health Service moved to recall the unused vaccines and to identify the cases that had developed from the vaccines. In 1935 too little was known about the poliomyelitis virus to do much more, and vaccination for poliomyelitis came to a halt for twenty years until fundamental knowledge could catch up. But the 1955 tragedy had been preceded by the most massive experiment in vaccination ever undertaken—and it had shown the vaccine used to be safe! Besides, the National Foundation for Infantile Paralysis, through the March of Dimes, had made the public acutely aware of the perils of poliomyelitis and the need for a vaccine. Obviously, the requirements set by the standards had not been rigorous enough. Modification of the process of inactivating poliomyelitis virus in the vaccine and revised requirements for the production of the vaccine[46] have resulted in vaccines that have caused no further trouble.

But the question arose as to why the tragedy should have occurred in the first place. The National Foundation and Dr. Jonas Salk were criticized for the fanfare of publicity that accompanied the release of the vaccine, for raising the public's expectation to a high pitch, and for refusing to admit that the original Salk formula for inactivation of the virus could have been inadequate.[47] The Public Health Service was criticized for releasing the vaccine without adequate testing on its part and for yielding to the pressures of the National Foundation. And Cutter Laboratories was also criticized for producing an unsafe vaccine, even though it had scrupulously followed the methods promulgated by Salk and prescribed by the Division of Biologics Standards. Also, the company was held to be legally responsible for the illnesses to the tune of over 3 million dollars.[48]

Perhaps the best lesson we can learn from this catastrophe is that no matter how much testing a drug has received under one method or stage of production, it must be tested rigorously when the methods or circumstances of production change. Then, too, we can relearn the age-old lesson that science and publicity mix about as well as oil and water. Finally, we must force ourselves to realize that in spite of optimal testing and the most rigorous surveillance, drugs will sometimes be unsafe. This is the price we pay for their many advantages. But we must be eternally vigilant to see that the price is as low as possible.

As we have already seen in the case of the recent poliomyelitis virus incident, the Division of Biologics Standards, being a part of the National Institutes of Health, is able to co-ordinate its work smoothly with other components of the Public Health Service; in this case, especially with the Communicable Disease Center. It also works closely with the National Institute of Allergy and Infectious Diseases in the production of vaccines. Although the division is not as intimately associated with the FDA, it appears that when administrative matters come up that require co-ordination, they are handled satisfactorily. Whether co-operation between the two agencies should be closer will be discussed after the work of the FDA has been considered.

. . . a modern American corporation understands well enough that it has a "constituency" to deal with. If its constituents—notably its buyers— are unsatisfied, they will go to the political state for solution.

—ADOLPH A. BERLE, JR.

Refusal to accept the inevitable shortcomings of any society is responsible for a good deal of what is best in political life.

—PETER F. DRUCKER

Truth, in the great practical concerns of life, is so much a question of the reconciling and combining of opposites, that very few have minds sufficiently capacious and impartial to make the adjustments with an approach to correctness, and it has to be made by the rough process of a struggle between combatants fighting under hostile banners.

—JOHN STUART MILL

11

The Food and Drug Administration: Present and Future

The process of testing drugs was compared in Chapter 4 to a series of sieves; the coarsest ones, the chemical, bacteriological, and animal tests, screen out a great many new drugs; these are followed by several progressively finer sieves as testing in humans passes through its several stages. It is the job of the federal FDA to supervise those sieves.

A new drug, as defined by federal law, is one that is not generally recognized among experts as safe and effective for the use proposed. Regulation by the FDA begins at the investigational stage. A new drug cannot be legally shipped in interstate commerce for testing in man until the sponsor (who is usually the manufacturer) submits to the FDA a Notice of Claimed Investigational Exemption for a New Drug (called an IND). On this form the sponsor must supply the quantitative composition of the drug, the methods used to insure its identity and uniformity, and the evidence for safety obtained from animal investigations. He must also state the plan of the proposed clinical studies and the qualifications of the clinical investigators. Clinical studies may proceed after this document is submitted unless the FDA believes that safety has not been adequately demonstrated in animals, but the FDA may stop clinical testing at any time upon evidence of probable toxicity or of violation of other provisions of the regulations.

Clinical tests are divided into three phases, as discussed in Chapter 4. Phases 1 and 2 are intensive studies on small numbers of patients or normal subjects, while Phase 3 comprises clinical trials on many patients. Investigators studying drugs in Phase 1 should be "thoroughly conversant with the action of drugs" according to the FDA, whereas in Phase 2 studies "should be conducted by clinicians familiar with the conditions to be treated, the drugs used in these conditions, and the methods of their evaluation."[1] Practicing physicians, whether specialists or non-specialists, may qualify to conduct Phase 3 studies. Investigators are required to keep adequate records, to make reports at least once a year to the sponsor (plus prompt reports of adverse reactions and immediate reports of dangerous ones), and to comply with the requirements for obtaining consent of persons receiving the drugs. It should be noted that the responsibility of the investigator is to the sponsor and not to the FDA, except when the investigator sponsors the drug himself.

After these studies are completed, the sponsor is ready to submit a New Drug Application (called an NDA). Approval of this application by the FDA is required before the drug may be marketed in interstate commerce. The NDA must contain the information obtained in tests on humans and the labeling the sponsor intends to use to identify and explain the use of the drug. Within 180 days the FDA must declare this application either approved, disapproved, or incomplete in one or more aspects (such as inadequate clinical data to support claims of efficacy or safety). If the sponsor disagrees with the judgment of the Bureau of Medicine of the FDA, he may request conferences with its staff; if he is still not in agreement, he may request an administrative hearing. If the ruling is against him there, he may appeal to the courts.

Now let us look at some of the significant problems that the FDA and the regulating parties have encountered under recent laws. The sparseness of our knowledge of the relationship of the actions of drugs in the lower animals to their actions in man has been mentioned in Chapter 3. The Drug Amendments Act of 1962 empowered the FDA to prohibit testing of a drug in humans until animal studies could predict that the drug could be given safely in man. But so much of the knowledge just was not there. One example is teratogenesis, the production of birth defects, by drugs.

The thalidomide tragedy alerted everyone to the potentiality of drugs for ruining the lives of the yet unborn. In most cases, however, we don't know the best animals to test to find out what drugs will do to human fetuses; we don't know what dose is best to give; we don't know when in pregnancy to give it.

Or take the adverse reactions that appear after prolonged use of a drug. As people live into the age groups in which they are likely to have chronic diseases, and as people suffering from chronic diseases are kept alive longer, prolonged treatment with drugs becomes an increasingly important problem. But our knowledge is not commensurate with the magnitude of the problem. As mentioned in Chapter 3, we are not always sure which animals to use to show the effects of long-term toxicity. We don't know whether three years' use in humans can be tested by three weeks' or three months' administration to an animal or whether we need to test the drug in animals for three years. FDA scientists found that certain drugs that acted on the nervous system sometimes damaged the eyes of animals, and some drugs used to prevent convulsions injured the eyes and glands of animals between the sixth and the twelfth month of continuous therapy.[2] Both groups of drugs are likely to be given to patients over periods of months or years.

The best the FDA can do under these circumstances is to set guidelines that follow the more conservative practices in present use. That these will seem extreme to some is a foregone conclusion. They can only be made less extreme if experiments show that less stringent tests will be equally predictive. This dilemma calls for doubled and quadrupled research by universities, the drug industry, and the FDA. Interest in such research has increased greatly in the past two or three years—a healthy outgrowth of the new law. For instance, in 1966 the Pharmaceutical Manufacturers Association published a survey of the relationship of studies on drugs in animals to studies in man.[3] The FDA was able to subscribe to most of the association's recommendations and incorporate them into its procedures.

In the early days of drug regulation the lack of chemical and pharmacological tests to determine the identity and purity of drugs hampered the enforcement of the laws. Scientists in industry, in universities, and in government moved into the vacuum and devised the tests. I am confident that in the next decade scientists will come up with methods for predicting toxicity of drugs in humans by the proper tests in animals. Meanwhile, energies must be channeled into new studies and not wasted on pointless recriminations.

Testing drugs in humans is much more complex than testing them in animals, as shown by the scarcity of rigorous and accurate studies in humans. For not only are studies in humans logistically more difficult than investigations in animals; they also introduce other considerations: the attitudes, feelings, and rights of the experimental subjects. This is one of the most explosive issues with which the FDA has had to deal.

The original Kefauver bill did not contain any provision for consent of the person in whom a new drug is tested. But, as mentioned in Chapter 10, an amendment to include the consent of the patient was introduced on the floor of the Senate[4] and was incorporated in the final version of the 1962 act. In interpreting this amendment, the FDA had to consider the problems inherent in obtaining information on the effect of new drugs on humans, the need for this information to protect the public, and the difficulty in interesting investigators in studying drugs in humans if added impediments were thrown in their way. On the other hand, it had to consider the right of every person to decide what will be done to his own body as recognized in the common law, in the wording of the new act, and in the comments of the legislators. For instance, Senator Carroll had said in the committee hearings: "I have great confidence in my doctors, but when they prescribe for me, I want them to tell me what they are doing, that is all. If they want to use me as a test, let them tell me. If I expect that for myself and my family, I expect that for every other American."[5]

After much deliberation the FDA proposed regulations requiring that the consent of persons on whom investigational drugs were used "primarily for the accumulation of scientific knowledge . . . must be obtained in all cases." For patients under treatment with investigational drugs consent was required "in all but exceptional cases." The exceptional cases were defined as those in which the investigator could not communicate with the patient or his representative or in which it would be contrary to the patient's welfare to obtain his consent, where "the communication of information to obtain consent would seriously affect the patient's well-being" in the physician's judgment. In obtaining consent the investigator must make known to the person who is to receive the drug "(taking into consideration such person's well-being and his ability to understand) the nature, expected duration, and purpose of the administration of said investigational drug; the method and means by which it is to be administered; the hazards involved; the existence of alternative forms of therapy, if any, and the beneficial effects upon his health or person that may possibly come from the administration of the investigational drug."[6]

The disputed problem of whether the consent should be in writing or not was compromised by requiring that for Phase 1 and Phase 2 investigations it should be written. In Phase 3 investigations the commissioner proposed that it be "the responsibility of investigators, taking into consideration the physical and mental state of the patient to decide when it is necessary or preferable to obtain consent in other than written form. When such written consent is not obtained, the investigator must obtain oral consent and record that fact in the medical record of the person receiving the drug."[7]

These regulations will unquestionably make it more difficult for investigators to obtain permission to try new drugs in some cases. An example would be the use of erythromycin for the treatment of pneumococcic pneumonia. When this drug was introduced, penicillin and the tetracyclines had already been shown to bring about prompt recovery in ninety-five of one hundred patients with pneumococcic pneumonia. In the infrequent case where the patient was hypersensitive to penicillin, a tetracycline could be used; and in the unusual instance where adverse reactions would prevent therapy with a tetracycline, penicillin could be used. It would be rare indeed to find a patient who could take neither. The only justification for the use of a third antibiotic in a patient who could be given one of the other two would be if the investigator honestly believed that the fatality rate from pneumonia could be lowered further by erythromycin than by the two antibiotics that had preceded it—a very unlikely possibility. How could he in good conscience ask a patient with pneumonia to take erythromycin? Yet it was important to test this third antibiotic in enough patients to determine its value because of the rare patient who might not be able to take the other two. Thus, it is possible that in conditions for which a therapeutic agent is available, strict adherence to the regulations may prevent us from finding a better one. How the medical profession will solve this dilemma remains to be seen.

Who is a properly qualified investigator? The Drug Amendments Act threw this prickly question into the hands of the FDA, which had never tried to handle it before. The FDA is touching it gently at present. It is not setting up criteria for investigators. For one thing, it is impossible to establish criteria that a majority of investigators will agree upon. Moreover, if such criteria could be established, they could not be met at this time, when most experts studying drugs have not had formal training in this field. Instead, the FDA has looked at the qualifications of the individual investigator in relation to the project he proposes to undertake, information that the sponsor must submit in an IND. Especially the FDA has looked at the reports of clinical investigators for flaws that indicate poor experimental design, inadequate supervision of experiments, and inaccurate or false observations. Following such a review, the agency has judged the clinical studies of a certain few physicians to be unsatisfactory.

In one case, an investigator has been indicted for furnishing false information to the FDA—for "rigged research," as Senator Humphrey called it.[8] In other less flagrant cases staff members of the FDA have pointed out to investigators that their work appeared to be carelessly done. Some have changed their methods of operating and have continued to study drugs for submission to the FDA; the investigations of others have been discontinued because the FDA has ruled them ineligible to receive investigational drugs.

More important than these few individual cases has been the publicity attendant upon them. This has alerted the drug companies, the medical profession, and the medical schools to the dangers to which investigators are exposed when their work is shoddy, slipshod, or dishonest. Perhaps specific criteria will eventually need to be evolved for those who investigate drugs in man, but the present system, by which the FDA determines the floor below which a clinical investigator cannot step and still study new drugs, seems to be working well. The challenge is then thrown to the medical profession to see how high it can elevate clinical investigators above that floor.

Whether as a result of the FDA's restraint or because investigators are learning to live with the new rules, complaints have diminished in recent months. Yet this does not necessarily mean that research has not been stifled. It is important that investigators in universities, hospitals, and research institutes continue to think about ways of introducing flexibility into the regulations. It is possible, for instance, that the FDA could be persuaded to turn over some of the responsibility to institutions themselves, if the institutions showed that they had properly functioning mechanisms for passing on and monitoring the use of investigational drugs. As mentioned in Chapter 4, the National Institutes of Health has shown that this system will work. This agency holds institutions strictly accountable for proper investigations in humans, at the same time allowing them to choose the methods by which they control these investigations.[9]

Although the Kefauver-Harris Amendments require the Department of Health, Education and Welfare to pass on the efficacy of drugs, they do not authorize that Department to refuse to approve an NDA for an effective drug on the basis that it is less effective than another drug. The legislative history of the bill shows that judgments of relative efficacy were definitely excluded. Senator Kefauver said, for instance: ". . . we are not talking about relative efficacy of one drug against the other. We are talking about a drug being efficacious for the uses for which it is intended and for which a claim is made."[10] But in diseases in which several drugs are effective, it is sometimes difficult to define efficacy except in comparison with other drugs. Before any specific treatment was available, thirty patients with pneumococcic pneumonia died out of every hundred. When sulfa drugs were given, only twelve patients died, but penicillin or the tetracyclines saved seven more. Should a sponsor of a penicillin or a tetracycline preparation make a claim for the superiority of his drug over sulfa drugs in pneumococcic pneumonia, the FDA would have to rule on it. Where the proof is so well documented as in pneumonia, the claim would be legitimate. But in hundreds of other cases the proof is not available; often no one has even attempted to get it. If a sponsor should make a claim of relative efficacy for his drug in such cases, it could not be accepted.

But in general, under the present laws the battles of relative efficacy will not be fought in the arena of a public agency because the evidence for many drugs is not sufficient for a conclusive decision. Questionable cases are left to the quasi-public agencies, such as the AMA Council on Drugs, the USP (*United States Pharmacopeia*), the NF (*National Formulary*), and the National Research Council, and to authors of textbooks and journal articles. This allows for differences of opinion, for champions of an idea to obtain new data and to present the facts to the medical profession, until the evidence in favor of one viewpoint is widely accepted.

A recurrent complaint of the drug companies is that the FDA requires them to submit a supplemental NDA whenever a change is made in the formula of a drug preparation, for instance in the flavoring of the solution in which the drug is contained. It is easy to see why this agency must be concerned with such changes when one recalls that it was the substance in which sulfanilamide was dissolved that caused the Elixir of Sulfanilamide disaster, described in Chapter 10. Certainly any formula that is changed must be proved to be safe, but when it comes to efficacy, it would be advantageous to all—manufacturer, FDA, and public—if simple tests were devised to show that the efficacy of the drug is the same as before.

A related issue is the FDA's refusal to use unpublished data gathered by one company without its permission in support of

the application of a second company for the sale of its brand of
the identical drug. This ruling, it can readily be seen, requires
duplication of animal and human experiments by the sponsors
of the different brands of the same drug. It also multiplies the
work of the FDA, since the agency must examine all the duplicate
data before approving the new brands. Yet to allow the use of
the original sponsor's data would be doing him a disservice in
the competitive market since he deserves a reward in the form
of "lead time" for his inventiveness in producing the drug first
and in devising the original tests.

Another reason why the FDA cannot accept the tests performed on one brand as proof of the efficacy of a different brand
is the doubt in many people's minds that different brands of the
same drug will be equally efficacious. The larger firms, which
are usually responsible for the innovations, have claimed that
different brands of the same preparation are not therapeutically
equivalent in humans. Some critics have assumed that there are
no essential differences. For instance, many witnesses who appeared before Senator Nelson's subcommittee implied that drugs
marketed under generic names were as effective as those
advertised under trade names.[11] The battle was mostly one of
words until Parke, Davis & Co. showed that Chloromycetin, its
brand of chloramphenicol, was absorbed more quickly and more
completely than the brands of three competitors.[12] The FDA
immediately moved to require each sponsor of chloramphenicol
to show by therapeutic trials that his brand was effective (as
Parke, Davis had done for Chloromycetin) or to prove that his
brand would produce blood levels similar to those produced by
Chloromycetin.[13] This action for the first time recognized the
reasonableness of assuming that the concentration of a drug in
the blood was related to its therapeutic efficacy.

For several decades the pharmaceutical companies have been
making more and more sophisticated preparations of drugs,
involving different coatings for capsules and tablets, different
particle sizes, different degrees of pressure in making tablets,
and various procedures intended to delay absorption from the
gastrointestinal tract. The *USP* and the *NF* made no move to

encompass these new departures, claiming that the companies would not submit data that would allow them to set up standards. Instead, they relied upon the disintegration time of a tablet or capsule, although this measurement does not necessarily correlate with the absorption of the drug into the blood.[14]

The variety of preparations marketed, and the wildness of some of the claims made, compounded the confusion and made regulatory action mandatory. Thus the FDA was forced to require a certain minimum of therapeutic efficacy for any brand of a drug. This was especially true where the drug was life-saving or was effective against a serious condition, where differences between brands were suspected, and where the differences were measurable.

It seems reasonable to assume that therapeutic effectiveness can be correlated with the concentration of the drug in the blood at intervals after ingestion or injection in humans (or in some other body fluid, such as urine, if that fluid is more related to the site of the infection). Yet data proving such a correlation are available for only a few drugs. Concentration of a drug in the blood or other fluid will have to serve as tentative evidence of therapeutic efficacy until we can either verify the relationship or have each brand tested for efficacy. This is in the public interest because it certifies that some evidence of effectiveness will be achieved by any brand of a drug that is allowed to be marketed. It enables a manufacturer of a superior brand to market it promptly, and it gives the manufacturers of other brands a target to shoot at in improving their products. But as *Drug Trade News* said in reporting a speech by Commissioner Goddard on biological availability of drugs: "There is a long, hard row to hoe before FDA comes near to its desired goal of being able to list the therapeutic equivalency or biological availability of thousands of drugs."[15] The Task Force on Prescription Drugs has predicted that adequate data on biological equivalency would be accumulated by 1971.[16] I believe that 1974 would be a more realistic date. But everyone would agree with the task force that obtaining this information should have a high priority.

Despite all obstacles and objections, the investigational drug program is moving ahead. The former director of the Bureau of Medicine reported that during the first four years after the Drug Amendments Act of 1962 became effective, 700 to 800 IND applications had been received each year, and about 2,000 to 2,500 products were under investigation at any one time.[17]

When the sponsor of a drug believes he has assembled enough information to show that a drug under investigation is safe and efficacious for the purposes for which he intends to make claims of efficacy, he submits an NDA. This must include the results of all animal and human studies, a description of the substances used in the manufacture, the methods of assaying the drug, the proposed labeling, and specified samples for testing in FDA laboratories.

Disparaging and derisive comments have been made by manufacturers about the mountains of data required for an NDA. Undoubtedly the records required are often voluminous; certainly it is hard to see how anything less than all of the data on a drug could be asked for, especially since some studies are so poorly done that the FDA has to scrutinize every detail. As Deputy Commissioner Rankin told industry representatives: "Some lousy work has been done in the name of science."[18]

In my opinion, much of this furor is merely static—the natural reaction of the regulated to strong regulation. The problem will be solved partly by well-designed studies of drugs, which will mean that a few studies can take the place of the many poor ones now reported. Other solutions are mechanical: uniform methods of reporting data, codification of information for reporting by computer systems, and agreement that certain portions will be summarized and certified as correct by the reporting sponsor. Any intentional or unintentional errors in these summaries would incur a heavy penalty and the revocation of the application.

A second storm center is the time required to process the NDA's. By law the FDA must act on an application within 180 days. If the application is approved, the drug can move in interstate commerce. If not, the sponsor may elect to obtain more data, or he may request a hearing, after which the commissioner must make a final decision.

The drug companies are naturally perturbed when they see the anticipated profits from a drug, which they have spent years developing, blocked in the narrow and congested channels of the FDA. A recent survey showed that the average time spent from the beginning of research on a drug until approval by the FDA was 6.8 years.[19] It is safe to say that on no problem has the Bureau of Medicine struggled harder than how to eliminate the "backlog" of NDA's. The need is for more manpower. But the private practice of medicine and the medical schools had been living on short rations of manpower for the past decade. Then, as a result of the 1962 law the drug industry, the FDA, and the Drug Division of the AMA suddenly wanted a larger share of an already sparse supply. The industry's higher salaries gave it an advantage over the FDA. At the same time, new rules for the testing of drugs were being made. The NDA's had become more voluminous, the standards had been set higher than ever before, and the staff of the FDA was distracted by the repeated excursions of congressional committees into their files, their activities, and even into their thoughts.

In the face of all this and the fact that the agency receives original new drug applications or resubmissions at the rate of one a day,[20] that it made any progress at all is praiseworthy, and that it was able to announce in June 1967 that the backlog of NDA's older than 180 days had been eliminated was remarkable.[21] Unfortunately, a small jam again developed after the doctors lent by the Public Health Service were released in July 1968. Also the backlog of supplemental NDA's is still monumental, and it sometimes takes longer than 180 days for a particular one to clear. When delays occur, there are good reasons: essential data are missing from the application, the data are not sufficient to prove safety and efficacy, there are questions about the validity of the observations, or the pros and cons are so closely balanced that a decision is difficult to make. If we look back on the decision whether or not to market thalidomide, several of these factors were present. The results of animal studies had raised a few nagging doubts. Then reports of nerve toxicity began to appear —just enough of them for Dr. Frances Kelsey to delay her decision. Then came the discovery of congenital malformations, and the drug was never marketed in the United States—to the great good fortune of the American public. For her devotion and good judgment Dr. Kelsey was given the Distinguished Federal Civilian Service Medal.[22]

Of course the record cannot always be so good as this. Many companies believe they have been unfairly treated because drugs that they consider worth-while and safe have not been approved rapidly. G. D. Searle & Co. complained that its brand of metronidazole, Flagyl, a drug for trichomonas infection of the vagina, still had not been cleared by the FDA nearly two years after the NDA had been filed, even though the AMA Council on Drugs had reported favorably upon it.[23]

On the contrary, a minor storm was loosed when amantadine was approved by the FDA. One of the first of the antiviral drugs, it has been shown to be effective in preventing only one type of influenza. Some virologists believe that it was approved too soon. They contended that its value was not sufficiently proved and its field of effectiveness was too narrow to justify its approval in the face of certain demonstrated toxic effects.[24] Such differences of opinion are found to follow many decisions of a regulatory commission. All we can expect is conscientious weighing of the evidence by the regulatory agency with consultation from outside experts in difficult cases, full disclosure of the agency's reasons when a decision is made, and aggressive action by the scientific community to get more evidence or to protest through the proper legal channels if they think the evidence is adequate.

One loud and recurrent criticism of the FDA by the drug companies has been that the professional people in the FDA lack the expertise to make the decisions thrust upon them. In view of the shortage of medical manpower, it is easy to see how both the drug companies and the FDA would have to settle at times for people with poorer qualifications than they would like. But if an incompetent lands in a drug company and makes mistakes, it merely means that the application will not be approved by the FDA; no harm will be done to patients, and the company can apply again when more data have been obtained. On the other hand, if a bungler is employed by the FDA and he holds up a drug that should be marketed, the agency is likely to be loudly berated by the drug company. If his mistake allows the sale of a worthless or dangerous drug, the whole world will hear about it.

What can the FDA do to improve this situation? Dr. R. Keith Cannan of the National Academy of Sciences reported to Senator Humphrey:

> *In the final analysis, the excellence of performance of FDA will rest upon the scientific competence, the intellectual power, and the professional integrity of the staff of the agency. Because the competition for men of high caliber and distinction in the medical world is severe, the strengthening of the staff will not easily be accomplished. Greater economic rewards are not enough. More important is the dissemination of a feeling of confidence that the agency is so administered as to encourage individual initiative in the development of policies and practices, active fellowship with the community of medical science, and a lively interest in investigative work. It is necessary to dispel the deadening impression that the agency is interested only in regulation. This aspect of the mission of FDA is, indeed, an impediment to intellectual excellence.*[25]

In testifying before Senator Humphrey's subcommittee in its hearings on interagency co-ordination in drug research and regulation in 1963, I made five recommendations for improving the professional work of the FDA: (1) a continuing advisory council; (2) continuing panels of experts as advisers; (3) better salaries; (4) more research by FDA physicians; and (5) closer co-operation with local universities.[26]

Requesting advice and assistance in decision-making from

experts from the scientific community outside the FDA is highly desirable, not only because it brings in other opinions, including those of the top authorities in a field, but also because it disseminates knowledge and ideas from and to the academic community. At first, after the passage of the 1962 act, the FDA seemed to drag its feet in appointing councils and committees. The Senate Committee on Government Operations claimed that there had been a nine-year delay after a Citizens Advisory Committee on the FDA first recommended the appointment of an advisory council and advisory committees.[27] By the end of 1967, however, a National Advisory Food and Drug Council, composed of representatives from the drug industry, the medical profession, and the public at large, had been formed to advise the commissioner, and an Advisory Board with representatives from the medical, dental, and veterinary professions was regularly meeting with the director of the Bureau of Medicine. In addition, nineteen committees had been formed to give advice on drugs for humans, one on veterinary medicine, two on foods, and one on research. This is an excellent start, but still more will be necessary to give the FDA the optimum help.

It has taken more time than was expected to form these committees because of problems of conflict of interest. Experts in a field are often already consultants for industry on a retaining fee, and some may own stock in pharmaceutical companies. I believe that the wisest course for any physician who is investigating drugs is to refrain from owning stock in a drug company. Although some may consider me too puritanical, I do not see how an investigator can be sure that his judgment may not be unconsciously colored by the fact that he shares, even though in a small way, the profits that could be affected by his decisions. On the other hand, the drug industry needs good men as consultants, and the liaison with the drug company is usually a two-way street. Important knowledge about new drugs and supplies of material for study often flow from the drug company to the medical school as a result of such a consultantship. It is obvious that if being a consultant to a drug company precludes advising the government, the drug industry and the FDA will compete for consultants, and the desire to render public service will vie with the more lucrative opportunities in the drug industry.[28] But many leading medical scientists are consultants for drug companies, and the FDA should not have to lose the benefit of their advice. The agency should be able to handle this possible conflict of interest by adopting the method used by the National Institutes of Health. Members of committees and boards of the FDA could absent themselves from the room when drugs sponsored by a company to which they are a consultant, or competitive drugs, are considered. The same system might be used if a member of a committee owned stock in a drug company.

The best way to elevate the scientific stature of the FDA is to increase the amount of research done in the agency. Research was an integral part of Wiley's original laboratory and has been a part of the agency's program ever since, although the tempo has varied depending upon the interest of the top officials in research and the generosity or stinginess of Congress in a particular year. Yet laboratories that test the identity and purity of drugs have been an intrinsic part of the FDA since the 1906 act, and while the amount of research still does not approach the ideal in the laboratories dealing with chemistry, pharmacology, and microbiology, it is woefully inadequate in the Bureau of Medicine. Once the 1962 law brought clinical investigation squarely within the scope of the FDA, it became important that the agency carry on research in this area also. It is axiomatic that clinical investigations should be judged by clinical investigators, but how are physicians in the FDA going to be clinical investigators unless they are working with human subjects or in laboratories on projects that are relevant to humans?

Some beginnings have been made. Physicians in the Bureau of Medicine have been encouraged to join the faculties of local medical schools and to participate in research programs with them, and in the first half of the 1968 fiscal year 77 physicians and dentists had done so, out of the total of 189 in the Bureau of Medicine.[29]

As of June 1968, eighteen contracts and agreements were in effect between the FDA and outside groups for research on drugs.

These varied in size from $6,600 to $1,188,000, the latter representing a contract with the Kaiser Foundation Research Institute to develop a system for monitoring drug reactions and for making a complete record of drug reactions among members of a large prepayment medical plan.[30]

But these are only a small part of what should be done. In addition to an enlarged program of contracts with outside agencies, the Bureau of Medicine needs its own laboratories and its own clinical facilities for the treatment of inpatients and outpatients, just as the Bureau of Science has laboratories in which approximately three hundred scientists conduct research in chemistry, pharmacology, microbiology, and other basic sciences as they relate to food and drugs.[31] The doctors in the Bureau of Medicine can be compared to doctors in the clinical departments of medical schools. Not until the turn of the century did these departments have their own laboratories, much later than the basic science departments. The clinical investigators in the FDA likewise need research facilities that their basic science colleagues already have. Planning for this should start now, so that eventually offices, laboratories, and clinical facilities could all be together in one complex.

The philosophy must permeate the FDA and the Department of Health, Education and Welfare that this agency must be a top scientific agency. It is easy to mouth these words, but to translate them into action means greatly increased numbers of physicians so that each may spend a larger part of his time in research; it means giving priority at times to a research problem over a regulatory problem when the administrators believe that in the long run solving the research problem will make for better regulation. As the vice president of the University of Chicago put it, the "policeman is becoming a professor."[32]

An alternate plan was proposed in June 1968 by Dr. James Shannon, director of the National Institutes of Health. He called for a top-level agency for the evaluation of drugs, presumably to be placed at the National Institutes of Health. The FDA would continue its regulatory function and continue to evaluate drugs from data supplied by drug companies, but when the data were conflicting or insufficient, it would ask the proposed evaluating agency to investigate the problem. This agency would be staffed with chemists, pharmacologists, pathologists, statisticians, and clinicians, and would not only conduct its own studies, but would also let contracts to other institutions for drug evaluation and award grants in areas basic to it.[33]

This plan has the advantage of bringing to bear the know-how and prestige of the National Institutes of Health. It has a prototype in the Division of Biologics Standards, which serves this function for serums, vaccines, and related problems. But the Division of Biologics Standards combines research and regulation, and there's the rub in Dr. Shannon's proposal. One recurring complaint about the FDA is that its doctors and scientists do not have the expertise to evaluate drugs properly, and another is that the "legal-minded" personnel of that agency dominate the decision-making. Under Dr. Shannon's proposed plan the doctors at the FDA would be "second-class citizens" in the eyes of their scientific colleagues and in the eyes of their regulatory-minded associates in the agency. Even though they would call upon the new agency for experimental studies, the interpretation and decision-making would be in the hands of the FDA, where it would be ideologically divorced from the influence of top-flight scientific minds.

The idea of a separate research agency is reminiscent of Harvey Wiley's attempt to make his Bureau of Chemistry of the Department of Agriculture the laboratory for the entire department—a plan that fell of its own weight, as the expanding needs of the Bureaus of Plant Industry, Forestry, Soils, Animal Industry, and others demanded a laboratory in each of these areas.[34]

As Dr. Charles May reminded a Senate subcommittee: "Scientific leadership is exercised only by working scientists truly occupied in the mainstreams of investigation. Membership in the scientific staff of the FDA cannot be made appealing simply by furnishing ringside seats to exciting research carried on in other arenas."[35] For these reasons, I believe it would be better if the scientific stature of the FDA were built up to the level of that developed at the National Institutes of Health under the able leadership of Dr. Shannon, so that collaboration between scientists and lawyers, between doctors and regulators, between the research-oriented and the service-oriented, could continue all along the line.

One group of drugs requires special consideration because they are biological rather than chemical substances and thus vary in potency. The public is protected best if the FDA itself is able to examine each individual batch of these drugs before it is marketed. The seed of this idea was planted in 1907 when manufacturers of coal-tar colors asked Dr. Wiley to certify those that were safe for use in foods and drugs. It was applied to drugs in 1941 when an amendment to the Federal Food, Drug, and Cosmetic Act required that the FDA approve each batch of insulin.[36]

In 1943 the FDA began testing samples of penicillin for the War Production Board, and in 1945, when penicillin was marketed, the Food and Drug Act was amended to include certification of batches of penicillin. Later other antibiotics were added. In 1960 an advisory committee to the Secretary of Health, Education and Welfare was appointed by the National Academy of Sciences to review the work of the FDA's Division of Antibiotics.[37] It recommended that all antibiotics used in man be certified, and this provision was included in the Drug Amendments Act of 1962.

Testing of these drugs has in the past been performed by different units of the FDA at different times. Since 1967 it has all been done in the National Center for Antibiotics and Insulin Analysis. As of May 1968 this center was responsible for certifying insulin and forty different antibiotics, of which there are hundreds of dosage forms.[38] During fiscal year 1968, 19,179 batches of antibiotics were submitted by drug firms for testing. Of these, 144 failed to meet proper standards.[39]

The sponsor of a new antibiotic is required to submit to the FDA an application that gives the components and composition of the drug, the methods used in its manufacture or fermentation, the tests used to assay its potency, and samples of the drug, as well as the results of clinical studies establishing its safety and efficacy. From these data and its own laboratory investigations the FDA prepares a monograph that establishes standards for the drug.

While the Center for Antibiotics and Insulin Analysis examines the drug in the laboratory, the Division of Anti-Infective Drugs of the Bureau of Medicine studies the evidence for its safety and efficacy when used as directed in the proposed labeling. Acting on the data submitted by the FDA laboratory as well as those submitted by the sponsor, this division accepts or rejects the New Drug Application and proposes the publication of a monograph in the Federal Register establishing standards, tests, and assays for the new drug. Insulin may be approved by the review of the data obtained in tests conducted in two independent laboratories.

Modern medicine continues to prove the truth of Hamlet's exclamation that:

> *. . . Diseases desperate grown*
> *By desperate appliance are relieved,*
> *Or not at all.*

In the treatment of cancer, certain severe infections, and other serious diseases and in the transplantation of organs, especially, the doctor must often use a potentially toxic drug. Most of the time such drugs are used in hospitals. But would it not be better to limit them entirely to hospitals, where laboratory tests would be available to follow the progress of the patient's disease and to monitor the toxic effects of the drug, and where the use of these drugs would come under the watchful eyes of the attending physician's colleagues? The FDA has required that labeling for a few drugs include this limitation. This should be done for more drugs, and some provision should be made to allow for administration of a drug to be continued after the patient leaves the hospital.

A further step would be to restrict the use of certain drugs to experts in particular fields. This explosive question was propounded in a speech by Commissioner Goddard in March 1967.[40] I would recommend that the FDA require that all highly toxic drugs that are effective in restricted areas, such as cancer therapy, be used only in hospitals. This would place them within the purview of the medical staff, which should then restrict their use to the members of the staff who are competent in that particular therapeutic area. Thus, government and practicing profession would be joining hands in improving therapy and preventing illnesses and deaths from drugs.

If new drugs pose problems for the FDA, older drugs create many more. Passing on the safety and efficacy of new drugs may be compared to certifying the purity of water in a city reservoir, while regulating old drugs is like guaranteeing that the water is still pure a hundred miles downstream after it has run past a dozen towns and cities. In view of the magnitude of the job it is not surprising that the program for older drugs is not as far along as that for new drugs. Yet much is already being done.

Drugs on the market that are being regulated by the FDA can be divided into four groups: (1) drugs approved for safety and efficacy under the provisions of the 1962 act; (2) those marketed under the 1938 Act, when safety was considered but efficacy was not; (3) the drugs still in use that were marketed before 1938, the sponsors of which were not required to prove either efficacy or safety; and (4) drugs that not only must be safe and efficacious before marketing but must be tested for potency (the antibiotics and insulin).

How does the FDA keep up with drugs after they have been marketed? For prescription drugs approved after June 1963, regulations require further reports from the sponsor on efficacy and adverse reactions coming to his notice, and any intended changes in labeling and advertising. Periodic reports must be made quarterly during the first year after approval of the drug, semiannually during the second year, and annually thereafter. Reports are required immediately in the case of unexplained failure in the activity of a drug, adverse reactions that are unusual because of severity or frequency, mix-ups in labeling, or chemical or bacterial contamination.

The reports required from sponsors are supplemented by reports of adverse reactions from individual physicians; groups such as the Council on Drugs of the AMA; regulatory agencies in other countries; hospitals, clinics, or medical schools under contract with the FDA to provide such information; and medical journals and books. The FDA also obtains information from pharmacists who observe mistakes in labeling or suspicious changes in the appearance of a drug. FDA inspectors make periodic visits to establishments where drugs are manufactured or packaged to detect irregularities; they also purchase drugs at intervals on the open market for testing in FDA laboratories.

This wide net of surveillance catches mistakes in manufacture and labeling as well as new facts that require action on individual drugs. From 1962 through 1967 approval was withdrawn for NDA's for seventeen drugs that had previously been approved. Eleven withdrawals were for serious adverse reactions, as in the case of triparanol (MER-29), which caused cataracts. Other approvals were withdrawn because of animal toxicity, lack of proof of efficacy, improper manufacturing practices, or unacceptable promotion.[41]

Surveillance procedures turn up general problems that call for solution. Obviously, the less surveillance has to deal with individual incidents and the more a single program can be extended to encompass a broad field, the more successful they will be. The FDA has already moved forward in two large areas: the reporting of adverse reactions and uniform labeling.

As mentioned in Chapter 9, the Council on Drugs of the AMA struggled with the reporting of adverse reactions for many years. As an educational venture, its program succeeded in keeping doctors alert to adverse reactions that were already known. But such reporting did not uncover any adverse reactions that had not been previously reported, nor did it detect the exact frequency of a reaction, since the number of persons who had received the drug was not known. In other words, the collector of such statistics had a numerator without a denominator.

The FDA tried the same method by contracting with hospitals to furnish data on all the adverse reactions to drugs that were observed in the hospital. It found that reporting was spotty, depending as it did upon the acuity and conscientiousness of the doctors with various degrees of interest.

Because of these inadequacies, the FDA tried another method. It awarded contracts to three hospitals to collect data on the drugs given to patients in the hospital and adverse reactions to them.[42] Hospitals lend themselves to such studies because all of the drugs come from a single pharmacy; also physicians' orders are more closely followed and records are more adequately kept than in the case of ambulatory patients. But the information obtained is limited by the relatively small number of patients observed and the fact that some drugs are used mostly in ambulatory patients. Similar surveys need to be made, therefore, on outpatients. All of these studies will provide needed information on the relative frequency of different adverse reactions to the same drug and of the same adverse reaction to different drugs; they should also uncover hitherto undetected adverse reactions.

The Drug Amendments Act of 1962 gave the FDA authority to initiate proceedings to prohibit the sale of a drug cleared for safety as a new drug under the act of 1938 if the agency believed there was a lack of substantial evidence of efficacy. A lag period of two years was allowed until October 10, 1964, so that the sponsors and the FDA might assemble any needed information.[43]

How was the FDA, short of staff, struggling to overcome the backlog of new drug applications that had accumulated in the two years since the act became effective, to take on this Herculean task? Commissioner Goddard's answer was a master stroke. He asked the National Academy of Sciences to make the evaluations. The academy, formed during the Civil War and designated by President Lincoln as an advisory board to the government in scientific matters, had grown in scope and prestige in the intervening years, especially during and after World War II. The academy accepted the task and placed it under the Drug Research Board of its working arm, the National Research Council.

This was a new departure in the evaluation of drugs. In taking this step the FDA leaned more heavily upon a private agency than ever before. True, it had accepted the standards established by the *USP* and the *NF*, but it had always done this after the fact. The *USP* and the *NF* had demonstrated that they could do the job expeditiously, thoroughly, and without bias; when they had proved this, their results were accepted. On the other hand, the National Research Council was being asked to take a major part in important decisions (although, it should be pointed out, not to make the final decisions) before it had demonstrated the capacity to do the job.

The organization for the study was set up promptly. Following the system so successfully used for many years by the *USP*, the National Research Council established twenty-seven (later thirty) panels of experts in different therapeutic areas. Some drugs had to be reviewed by several panels because they had several different therapeutic uses, one drug by fifteen different panels.

The sponsors of the drugs were required to submit information identifying the product and, if they desired, other information pertinent to an evaluation of efficacy. This was turned over to the panels, who combined it with data from the files of the FDA, from the literature, from conversations with colleagues, and from their personal experience. Conflict of interest was handled by having members of panels absent themselves from any deliberations in which a company with which they had close relationships might have an interest. In their reports the panels classified the drugs as "effective," "probably effective (requiring additional evidence before it can be placed in the first category)," "possibly effective," "ineffective," and in an additional category added by the panels themselves, "effective, but with qualifications." The last group might include, for example, a preparation for iron deficiency anemia that contained, in addition to iron, a trace element of another substance for which there was no evidence of effectiveness in anemia. The panel might rule that the preparation was effective in anemia as claimed, with the stipulation that it contained a trace element that appeared to have no therapeutic value.

During the period between the acts of 1938 and 1962, it is estimated that NDA's were approved for more than 7,000 drug preparations for humans, of which 2,824 sets of preparations (or approximately 3,700, counting all dosage forms) were being marketed at the time the study by the academy got underway. These were sponsored by 237 firms. It is estimated that for every drug for which an NDA was on file, about five others, which represented duplications, were being marketed by companies who had never submitted an NDA. This means that over 20,000 drug preparations will be affected by the National Research Council's drug efficacy review.[44]

By April 1969 the National Research Council had reported on all of the drug preparations. Most of these were still under consideration by the FDA, although the agency had begun to act on them. On January 23, 1968, Commissioner Goddard published the first notice on any of these drugs; he stated that there was no evidence that the bioflavinoids (discussed in Chapter 4) were effective for use in man in any condition,[45] and that an informal hearing on the subject would be held as a first move toward withdrawing approval of these drugs. Since then, the FDA has disapproved claims for a number of other drugs in conformity with recommendations by the National Research Council.

Considering the prestige of the National Academy of Sciences, considering the elaborate procedure that had been devised to make a thorough study of the information available on each drug investigated, considering that the drug industry had consistently clamored for an "unbiased" group to pass judgment on drugs, considering that the committee selecting the members of the panels contained representatives from industry as well as from the academic community and the medical profession, many people expected that the sponsoring companies would abide by the recommendations of the National Research Council and the actions of the FDA based on them. But, apparently, this is not to be. The FDA's decision on the bioflavinoids has been challenged, possibly because these compounds represent a multi-million-dollar market,[46] and one lawyer has predicted that the FDA will be faced with over a hundred hearings in the near future.[47]

Thus, while the mechanics of the most radical departure from previous methods of government regulation worked well, the outcome is still uncertain. All the evidence points toward a fair and complete assessment of the information on the drugs evaluated. The sponsor of each drug has received the report of the council's panel on the drugs he sponsored. This may be followed by informal conferences with FDA officials and a formal hearing if desired. If he is still not satisfied, the case may be carried to the courts.

In spite of the many new drugs that have been and still are being introduced, some are still used that were available before the 1938 act, at which time the FDA began clearing new drugs. The safety and efficacy of these drugs should by now have been established, and the doctors prescribing them should be well informed about them. Yet, as mentioned in Chapter 4, we are continually finding new facts about such drugs as aspirin and digitalis, which have been in common use for more than fifty years, and we must assume that new facts will be encountered concerning other established drugs, which will call for change in usage or complete abandonment. In such cases, one hopes that the message will reach the practicing doctors. But it is obvious that an information gap is unavoidable when we realize that there is no authoritative list of all the drugs now available on the market, not even at the FDA! If we needed more testimony in favor of the newer provisions for registration and inspection of all drug firms and all applications for new drugs, this fact should speak eloquently for such provisions.

Labeling includes everything from the package insert (or stuffer, as it has been somewhat jocularly called) to pamphlets and books promoted or distributed by a sponsor concerning drugs that it sells. Under regulations promulgated in 1961, the labeling must give full and adequate disclosure of the important information available about the identity, actions, uses, effectiveness, and the possible adverse effects of a drug; it must be neither false nor misleading, and the regimen recommended in the labeling must be such that it can be carried out safely in the dosage recommended.

Historically, the label arose as an attempt by the seller to inform his customer what was in a package and to persuade him to buy it. When the labels attached to the boxes or bottles were too small for all the vendor wanted to say, he began to put circulars in the containers. This enabled him to say a lot more, and much of it was in superlatives.

The advent of laws requiring that labeling contain true information on safety and efficacy demanded a shift in emphasis from huckstering to education. This shift is by no means complete today. It is very much in flux—and it has created problems. The initiative is with the sponsor of the drug, who devises the labeling and submits it to the FDA as a part of the NDA. The FDA informs the sponsor of any criticisms or suggested modifications, and the sponsor either changes the labeling to conform or seeks a compromise. Clearly, the label and the pamphlet are commercial documents intended primarily to identify and sell a drug. Although the FDA often requires drastic changes from the original draft, labeling still tends to have a commercial flavor. Also, in spite of the fact that the FDA has approved the labeling, the law does not permit the sponsor to make any statement to that effect.

The FDA has ruled that whenever a sponsor initiates a change in the labeling, the entire package insert should be reviewed. Since this may mean considerable work for the sponsors, they are obviously loath to make changes. For this reason and because of the sheer size of the job of keeping all of the facts up to date, much of the labeling for drugs already on the market is far behind present-day knowledge. Sometimes the FDA itself initiates a change, but in the light of all the other monitoring it has to do, this doesn't happen as often as it should.

Of course, the labeling for many drugs will be updated when the recommendations of the National Research Council are implemented.

Labeling for a brand of drug sold by one company may differ greatly from the labeling for another company's brand of the same drug. Or labeling for drugs of closely related chemical structure and clinical effectiveness may read in such a way that each drug seems to be totally unrelated to the other. Such discrepancies have sparked a movement toward uniform labeling. Under this system officials of the FDA and representatives of the companies marketing a particular group of drugs meet and hammer out uniform wording for the entire group. An advisory committee of outside scientists may participate in the discussions. Sometimes agreement is reached; in other cases the FDA has to make a decision that it considers to be in the public interest, in spite of contrary opinions of a minority or even a majority of the sponsors.

Two lines of procedure are open at this point: the FDA may establish unofficial guidelines for writing labeling for this class of drugs. These guidelines are furnished to the sponsor of a new drug or of an established drug when the need for revised labeling arises. This method has been used in the case of the thiazide diuretics, the corticosteroids, and the phenothiazines. Alternatively, the FDA may issue regulations covering uniform labeling, as was done in the case of the coronary vasodilating drugs. If the co-operation of the drug industry can be obtained, the former method is to be preferred to the rigidity of the latter.

In a more controversial field involving a more widely used group of drugs, the oral contraceptives, the FDA went one step farther. Not only did it devise a format for uniform labeling of these drugs, but it sent a copy of this form to every doctor so that he could be informed especially about the danger of thrombophlebitis in women taking these drugs. (Thromboplebitis is the development of a clot in a vein, usually a vein in the leg or thigh. It may be dangerous because a part of the clot may break off and lodge in an artery that supplies blood to a vital organ.) Slight though the danger is—only 47 cases in 100,000 women taking contraceptive drugs as compared with 5 cases in a similar number of women not using them—the widespread use of what has come to be called "the Pill" made it mandatory that doctors should be told promptly about this adverse effect.[48]

The movement toward uniform labeling is only starting. It needs to be extended until all classes of drugs are included, because it is one way to simplify the tangled mass of information that reaches the physician.

As mentioned in Chapter 4, information about drugs intended for use in young children and pregnant women is especially scarce. I have already alluded to the difficulty, often impossibility, of translating from animals to humans the results of experiments on injury to the offspring resulting from drugs given to mothers. Investigators are necessarily loath to give a new drug to pregnant women until a large number of other persons have first taken the drug without ill effect. Should the labeling, then, forbid the use of the drug in pregnant women? This would place in a legally untenable position the physician who felt impelled to use the drug in a seriously ill pregnant woman in whom other measures had been ineffective. It is better for the labeling to state that the drug has not received sufficient trial in pregnant women so that safety for the fetus can be assured. The decision whether to use the drug in a pregnant woman in a serious case would then be left to the patient's doctor.

On the other hand, when a drug is suspected of causing birth defects, more positive action must be taken. The FDA met this problem in the case of the antinauseant drugs meclizine, cyclizine, and chlorcyclizine by requiring that when those drugs were sold without prescription over the counter, they should bear a warning statement that they should not be used by women who were pregnant or might possibly become pregnant. For prescription drugs in this group the FDA required a statement calling attention to adverse effects of the drug on the offspring of animals, voicing the suspicion that it might possess a potential for adverse effects in the human fetus and stating that there is no substantial evidence that it is beneficial in the nausea and vomiting of pregnancy.[49]

What to put on the labels regarding the doses of drugs that should be given to children also poses a problem. Here the bottleneck is the lack of children to test. Most drugs are evaluated initially in adults, and the dosages established for them. These dosages cannot be directly transposed to children on the basis of relative age or weight or other criteria because children sometimes metabolize a drug entirely differently from adults; one fourth of the adult dose given to a child weighing one fourth as much as the average adult might be too little to be effective or so much as to be toxic. Thus drugs must be tested in children before being recommended for children. But a child cannot legally give consent for such human experimentation, and parents are naturally reluctant to do so. Consequently, the dosages of many drugs have not been established for children, and the labels must bear a statement to this effect. The national pediatric societies are actively studying the problem of obtaining more testing of drugs in children; let us hope they come up soon with an answer.

Before the 1962 act the FDA took the position that its duties related entirely to the sponsors of drugs. Contacts with the practicing doctor are a new experience—an experience that the agency has found to be prickly with problems. It has required drug companies to send warning letters to doctors (familiarly called "Dear Doctor letters") about serious adverse effects of a drug that have come to light, and on occasion the FDA itself has sent such a letter. Both types of letters are picked up by the general news media and may generate unfavorable publicity for the drug and its sponsor.

No one seems to know whether doctors read these letters or, if they read them, whether they remember them or keep them on file or, if they remember or refer to them, whether they adhere to them. If these letters do, in fact, change doctors' actions, are the letters sent by the FDA more influential than those sent by a drug company? Surely we should be finding out what effect these letters have. I hope that investigators in universities will undertake the task. If not, the FDA should do it.

Meanwhile, the labeling, especially the package insert, remains the one source of information about a drug approved by the FDA. Thus it is easy to see how the labeling is coming to represent in some people's minds the legal standard that defines the proper use of a drug and from which the practitioner deviates at his peril. If he gives the drug in a different dosage or for different reasons than the label recommends, the burden of proof may be on him to show that he had good reason to do so. In one case a package insert was used as testimony in court against a dentist,[50] although in a later case the Massachusetts Supreme Court decided that "the package insert is no more and no less important than any other medical reference available to the physician."[51] It is important that the FDA avoid the requirement of rigid dosage regimens and mandatory conditions for the use of a drug, since these place the doctor in a strait jacket in treating his patients. Recently there has been some relaxation in these areas, but each new label should be looked at critically by the FDA and outside groups, preferably before the final decision is made. Surveillance of the FDA's actions in this regard is an important responsibility for the AMA.

The federal laws give the FDA no direct jurisdiction over a physician's actions. Once a drug is approved for sale, the physician prescribing it is not restricted to the uses listed in the labeling. If he prescribes a drug for some purpose not specified in the labeling, however, he should be sure that his reasons are defensible, since he might be held liable in a civil suit in case the results were unsatisfactory. Also, if a physician is using a drug for conditions not as yet approved by the FDA for the purpose of eventually obtaining such approval or in collaboration with a drug firm, someone, either the drug firm or the physician, is required to submit an IND.

The FDA also believes that its obligation to inform physicians of serious adverse effects of a drug may at times require it to call attention to authoritative sources of information, such as textbooks, that do not coincide with the approved labeling for the drug. Acting under this interpretation, the FDA took an unprecedented step in 1967, when it found that the dose of a drug used to treat intestinal parasites, recommended in a widely read book on therapeutics, was two to four times that recommended in the package insert. Because children had died, apparently as a result of administration of the drug, the agency asked the publisher of the book to state that the dose in the textbook was higher than the dose shown in the approved labeling. When the author was approached, he chose instead to remove all reference to the drug. Had the publisher not complied, the FDA would have had the legal right to inform all of the physicians in the country that an unsafe dose was being recommended, and of course this would have had damaging effects upon the reputation of the book.

In protesting this action, the editor of *Clinical Pharmacology and Therapeutics* gave three reasons why the label could not be considered a standard to be slavishly followed by authors of textbooks: (1) A drug must be in active use for some time—he suggested approximately five years—before even the experts can be sure about its dosage under most conditions, and there must be free exchange of information and opinion during that period. (2) The FDA does not have a corner on the expert opinion of the country. A substantial number of experts may disagree with its opinions as to dosage. (3) The labeling is frequently not up to date. The editorial concluded: "To hold scientists and physicians in jeopardy if they dare disagree publicly with the FDA is against all the canons of science and scholarship. In our opinion, it is in the worst interests of our nation's *health*, it is a barrier to *education*, and it is for no one's *welfare*. The new policy comes strangely from an agency of the United States Department of Health, Education, and Welfare."[52]

In defense of the FDA's action, Dr. Ley claimed that the FDA had "the responsibility to withdraw approval or issue warnings for drugs presenting a hazard to health." Since "the unqualified dosage recommendations carried in the table of the textbook could lead to further unnecessary deaths," the FDA chose to make its suggestion to the publishers rather than inform physicians that the dose recommended in the package insert was lower than that given in the textbook.[53] He made a distinction between a textbook that is generally considered to represent standard medical practice and books and articles that present individual opinions and controversial views. The FDA also made the point that it cannot compel the publisher to change something in his book. Yet it is clear that a threat to warn doctors of a putative error would in fact be compulsion.

Later Julius Hauser of the FDA denied that the agency had any intention of attempting the censorship of medical journals, medical textbooks, or any other private medical publications.[54] But it appears to me that without intending it, that is what the agency managed to do. Let us hope that the action has alerted publishers and authors sufficiently to the significance of the dosages recommended in textbooks that the incident will never have to be repeated.

Among the methods of getting information on drugs to the physician, one seems to be attracting the most attention, a compendium that would include all the drugs available in this country and important facts pertaining to them. A compendium is being advocated for informative and for economic reasons. The Task Force on Prescription Drugs recommended:

"The Secretary of Health, Education, and Welfare should be authorized to publish and distribute a drug compendium listing all lawfully available prescription drugs, including such information as available dosage forms, clinical effects, indications and contraindications for use, and methods of administration, together with price information on each listed product."[55]

Everyone agrees that the practicing physician seldom sees the package insert unless he requests a copy of it either from a pharmacist or from the sponsor, unless it is mailed to him along with an advertisement or a drug sample, or unless he purchases the drug himself for dispensing or injecting. Not many physicians maintain files of package inserts, although pharmacists are beginning to do this for purposes of answering doctors' inquiries.

The books that are now available to the doctor do not give him all the information he needs. *New Drugs*, published by the

AMA, comes nearest to it, but it contains only those drugs introduced in the past ten years; it ignores mixtures, of which there are many; it does not state the dosage forms available; and it sometimes is criticized for being "weasel-worded"—for not stating forthrightly that the evidence does not justify a claim that is being made for a drug. Textbooks on therapeutics are less authoritative since they usually represent the opinion of only one man; they do not pretend to cover all drugs, and they are not kept up to date as a reference book must be. The *Physician's Desk Reference*, as would be expected from the fact that it is distributed without charge to all physicians, is essentially a series of advertisements. In the indexes producers' and trade names are played up, generic names are played down. Some companies and some products are not represented at all. Nevertheless, it does contain the most nearly complete list of drugs readily available to the physician, and because the FDA now requires that all statements conform to the approved labeling, it is a valuable source of information on adverse reactions and dosages. The *USP* (*The United States Pharmacopeia*) and the *NF* (*The National Formulary*) contain nothing of immediate value to the physician except the names of drugs selected as the best ones in various fields and the usual doses; consequently, they are not used by him.

Thus there is a void that could be filled by an up-to-date listing of all drugs moving in interstate commerce, including mixtures, indexed by generic and trade names; the diseases and symptoms for which they would be used; and information on adverse reactions, dosage forms, and sponsors. Unfortunately, the informational uses of such a book have been intertwined with the economic aims by many of its advocates. The urge to cut the costs of medical care has generated a campaign to per-suade the doctor to prescribe drugs by generic name. Such a purpose would be highly served by a handy listing of the prices of drugs, either along with other information about them or in a supplement. This was the recommendation of President Johnson in his special message to Congress on health.[56]

The drug industry has poured cold water on the compendium

concept, probably because it is an economic threat, although the reasons given are its unwieldy size, the difficulty of being sure that it would be unbiased, and keeping it up to date.[57] The industry may also have objected because it has been suggested that it finance a free copy for every doctor, since a complete compendium could replace package inserts.

From my experience in the practice of medicine, as a teacher of medical students and house officers, and as a former chairman of the Council on Drugs of the AMA, I strongly believe that the information on drugs available at the physician's elbow at the moment he needs it is woefully deficient, and while a national system of computerized information such as has been advocated is greatly to be desired, it will not serve the purpose of on-the-spot reference for the emergency and for the great preponderance of small facts that need looking up or verifying in the doctor's day-to-day work.

Can the doctor's needs be served best by the kind of compendium advocated by the FDA? To answer this we should take a look at what has been done in the past. When a book of standards for drugs was needed, a private agency, the United States Pharmacopeial Convention, was formed to produce it. But the *USP* includes standards for only a blue-ribbon list of drugs— those selected by experts as the best to use in practice. Some doctors used other drugs, and the *NF* was begun so as to include the best of these. At first most of the drugs eliminated from the *USP* were therapeutically ineffective or decidedly inferior to other drugs, but as the number of drugs multiplied, many just-as-good preparations were to be found in the *NF*.

Also, the *USP* was published at intervals of ten (later five) years. The AMA stepped into the breach with *NNR* (*New and Nonofficial Remedies*), later *NND* (*New and Nonofficial Drugs*), which was published each year and listed new drugs not yet in the *USP* or the *NF*.

Finally, the early mixtures often contained several worthless ingredients and only one effective drug (or none at all). But today many mixtures on the market contain two or three effective drugs. Such mixtures are widely advertised to physicians, they are extensively prescribed, and they cannot be ignored. Yet, with only a few exceptions, they are not included in the *USP*, the *NF*, or *New Drugs*. Since private groups have not kept up with the times and since the new laws have thrust this hot potato into the hands of the FDA, this agency naturally would embrace a solution that at one sweep would make up for the information deficit of the past half-century.

But just because the information gap is enormous, a *tour de force* to fill it is likely to result in a book that may be more authoritarian than authoritative and more conforming than path-finding. Instead, I would encourage the AMA to speed the completion of its proposed book, *ADE* (*AMA Drug Evaluations*) and to include information on the different brands and their prices. This book will be an authoritative source of information made by groups of experts, on the basis of information supplied by pharmaceutical companies, the package inserts, a review of the scientific literature, and their personal experiences. It will be of manageable size and it will compare drugs in the same class with one another. Other groups are capable of publishing an authoritative compendium and should be challenged to do so.

If *ADE* meets the needs of physicians and of the regulatory agencies, it may be recognized by the FDA as a replacement for the package inserts. Or the FDA may recognize, instead or in addition, a compendium published by some other group. The problem of financing the book and making sure that every doctor sees it can be solved by requiring that every licensed practitioner own a copy, just as many states require that each pharmacist have a copy of the *USP* and the *NF*.

Mechanisms of collection and storage of information, such as those centered at the National Library of Medicine, can and should be perfected as the most comprehensive and up-to-the-minute source of information that could be called upon for unusual, urgent, and complicated cases. These recommendations do not deliver the Goddess of Drug Information full-grown from the forehead of Zeus. But in a democracy we should have no Zeus, and mortal life requires man to fulfill his function by growth rather than by fiat.

In Chapter 7 I took up the criticisms of the advertising of drugs and the defense made by the drug industry, and concluded that drastic improvements were needed, many of which would follow now that the FDA is empowered to regulate advertising. Since this regulation had to rest upon a proper evaluation of drugs, that agency, after the passage of the 1962 act, was forced to tool up to evaluate claims of efficacy and to improve the reporting of adverse reactions before tackling advertising. By October 1963, however, the FDA had issued regulations on advertising and had conferred with representatives of firms that objected to them.[58] The act and the regulations laid down several requirements: (1) The established name (i.e. the generic name) should be printed in letters at least half as prominent as the proprietary name and should accompany the proprietary name each time that was featured. (2) A brief summary of side effects, contraindications, and effectiveness should be included in any advertisements that purported to give the dosages of a drug or to tell under what conditions it should be used. (Other advertisements that do not give dosages or recommend uses are called "reminder ads.") (3) A fair balance should be made in presenting the information on effectiveness and that on side effects and contraindications. (4) Recommendations or suggested uses in advertisements should be confined to those contained in labeling permitted by the FDA in the New Drug Application or its supplement. (5) Preclearance of advertisements by the FDA is not required unless a sponsor has been notified by the FDA to correct the advertising of a drug and has failed to do so.[59]

In spite of protests from representatives of the drug industry over some of the details of the regulations, advertisements for drugs in medical journals had improved greatly by the beginning of 1964. Yet some were as unreliable and misleading as ever.[60] Commissioner Goddard told the Pharmaceutical Manufacturers Association that in 1965 the small staff of the FDA that was monitoring advertisements had passed on to the Bureau of Regulatory Compliance complaints involving nearly one-third of the firms who were members of that association. He continued: "Some advertising cases have been quite abusive of regulations.

They have trumpeted results of favorable research and have not mentioned unfavorable research; they have puffed up what was insignificant clinical evidence; they have substituted emotional appeals for scientific ones."[61]

The FDA mounted an aggressive campaign to bring violators to bay. At first it followed the practice of holding a conference with a firm when one of its advertisements appeared to be violating regulations. Later, it began to issue a formal citation to a company asking that it show cause why the misbranding of a drug resulting from improper advertising should not be referred to the Department of Justice for prosecution. When these measures did not bring sufficient improvement in drug advertising, the FDA took a more drastic step; it seized shipments of drugs that had been improperly advertised. In such a case, the sponsor may elect not to contest, or he may defend his position in court; if he wins, the advertisement need not be changed. More important, adverse publicity usually forces the sponsor to change the advertisement. In fact, the publicity from these seizures was enough to bring howls of outrage from the drug industry and to cause two leading companies to threaten to withdraw all their advertisements from medical journals.[62]

Whether because the agency believed the method of seizure was too extreme or because it decided that another method might get corrective information to the doctors more rapidly, it changed its policy and required a drug company to send a letter to all of the licensed practitioners in the United States stating that the FDA considered a particular advertisement misleading and giving the correct facts. In the eighteen months ending in January 1969, it directed that twenty-nine letters be sent in connection with advertisements in journals or in the *Physicians' Desk Reference*.[63]

One further step has been taken by the FDA. Since representatives of the drug and advertising industries had complained that the regulations were not specific enough,[64] the FDA officials devised more specific rules after consultation with industry representatives. Among other provisions, they enumerated twenty specific conditions in which an advertisement would be considered "false, lacking in fair balance, or otherwise misleading." These ranged all the way from the use of quotations from medical authorities and publications to the proper use of statistical data.[65]

The drug industry has not accepted these restraints without protest. The Pharmaceutical Manufacturers Association called many of the rules "unreasonable, arbitrary and capricious."[66] Yet I believe that an examination of advertisements in medical journals today will convince a careful reader that they are greatly improved over those appearing before 1962. Some idea of the change can be obtained by comparing advertisements for identical drugs published at approximately the same time in the *British Medical Journal* and the American edition of the *Lancet*. Although the latter is also a British publication, the advertisements in the American edition have to comply with requirements of the FDA. An advertisement for Aldomet, Merck Sharp & Dohme's trade name for methyldopa, used to treat high blood pressure, in the *British Medical Journal* on June 29, 1968, consisted of a picture, some headlines, and a few lines of text recommending uses for the drug. Four lines were quoted from an article favorable to methyldopa.

In contrast, the advertisement in the American edition of the *Lancet* on May 4, 1968, showed a full-page picture of the blood vessels of the kidney. A second page consisted mostly of text, 25 per cent of which was devoted to side effects and 40 per cent to precautions. The balance achieved in the second advertisement pointed up the lack of it in the first, in which the text was confined to the virtues of the drug, adverse reactions were not mentioned, only one favorable article was quoted, and no attempt was made to compare this with other articles. The generic name of the drug in the first article was about one twentieth the size of the trade name and could hardly be read; in the American advertisement it was half the size of the trade name.

Of course, the constantly recurring question is still with us: how much is the practicing physician affected by the change in the advertisements? How much does he read them? This subject cries for investigation; but until such studies are made, we can at least be sure that if the physician does read today's advertisements, he will get a more balanced picture of the advantages and disadvantages of the drug advertised.

The promotion of a drug revolves around a central theme; this is carried through the advertising in all media—not only the medical journals, but also direct mailings, films, and the sales patter of the detail men. All of these come within the purview of the FDA. It has ruled that it has jurisdiction over films, except those that are made for purely educational purposes. Direct mailings are harder to regulate because of their large number. Surveillance over detail men is almost impossible, but not entirely so. The written material given by a firm to its detail men as the basis for their talks with physicians is available to the FDA, and physicians can report to the FDA when detail men have given them misleading or incorrect information.

All in all, this first industry-wide experiment in the strict regulation of advertising is an enormous job, and as the FDA has repeatedly contended, the small force at its disposal cannot do it adequately. The co-operation of the medical profession, the editors of medical journals, and the drug companies is also needed. Physicians, by being alert to the requirements laid down for advertising, can perform a public service by reporting to the FDA when advertisements reaching them in any of the media do not comply with regulations. Editors of the better medical journals have striven for a long time to make sure that the advertisements in their publications are factual, in good taste, and not misleading. Now they have help from the federal government, and together the two groups can do the job better than ever. Besides, some advertisements have shown a decided lack of taste. Why the naked figure of the female should be relevant to so many drugs remains a mystery. Since the FDA does not (and should not) attempt to be a judge of taste, the responsibility falls upon the editors of the journals. It is time that they realize (if the drug companies do not) that such practices belittle the professionalism of the very persons they are intended to influence.

Finally, drug companies now have the opportunity to make their advertisements factual and informative, to render a true service to the practicing physician and, through him, to the public. In the past, those firms that hewed to the line more rigorously were haunted by the fear that the companies who were "stuffing the ears of men with false reports" would steal business away from them by their sharp practices, and no doubt they did. Now the company with a consistently honest program of advertising should reap the benefits of it because it will not have the bother, the delay, and the publicity attendant upon censure by the FDA.

An English critic wrote in 1890: "Suppose a dozen people are in a small room. Two begin to talk to each other at the top of their voices. The others must either give up conversation or shout also. The result is that no one hears as well as before and that comfort is at an end. So it is with advertising. . . ."[67]

Now perhaps we are beginning to reverse the process!

A regulatory agency in a democracy must walk the thin line between authoritarianism and laxity, between rigidity and flexibility, between the interests of the individual and the welfare of the public. These different and sometimes opposed interests must be safeguarded by a legal system that assures each party his "day in court." If the FDA refuses to approve a New Drug Application or withdraws its approval and if the differences have not been resolved in informal conferences, the sponsor can request an administrative hearing at which testimony is taken from both parties before a hearing examiner. A decision is then made by the commissioner of Food and Drugs on the basis of the evidence. If the decision is in the sponsor's favor, it is final; if against the sponsor, the case can be reviewed by the court of appeals, and if another adverse decision results, the Supreme Court may review it.

A regulated industry is constrained to imitate the ballplayer who argues with the umpire. It may not expect to change the announced decision but hopes that the protest will affect the next decision. The strategy of a regulated industry is to keep the pressure on the regulator, to seek for persons or procedures that are likely to give way, and to push persistently in these spots. Sometimes this persistency becomes harassment, as was the case when Dr. Kelsey and her superiors received fifty contacts in the form of visits and telephone calls from the sponsor when the

FDA refused to approve thalidomide.[68] A certain amount of persistence is natural, some excess in zeal is excusable. But when company doctors, sales managers, lawyers, and executives descend upon the doctors of the FDA in wave after wave, time and energy are wasted on both sides.

FDA-industry relations have been debated since the passage of the first food and drug law. Should the sole function of the FDA be to punish wrongdoers? Harvey Wiley thought so and accused his superiors and his successors of being soft on industry. Since his day none of the commissioners of food and drugs have taken such a hard line, although some have at times spoken sharply to industry officials as did Commissioner Goddard when he said: "Too many drug manufacturers may well have obscured the prime mission of their industry: to help people get well."[69]

Even the most contentious of congressional critics have not gone so far as Dr. Wiley. Some observers believed that Commissioner Larrick, like Richard II,

> . . . *basely yielded upon compromise*
> *That which his noble ancestors achieved with blows."*

And the *Wall Street Journal* claimed that "Dr. Goddard's unquestioned contribution has been to alter the FDA's public image from pro-industry pal under his predecessor . . . to rigorous consumer protector."[70] Perhaps co-operation with the drug industry tarnished the image of the FDA in some eyes, but the same people criticized the FDA's small staff and the consequent difficulty in getting its job done. If the agency had not depended upon some self-regulation by the drug companies, it would either have been bogged down in a morass of trivia, or it would have become a huge juggernaut prepared to crush everything in its path. In my opinion Commissioner Larrick's testimony before a subcommittee of the House of Representatives states an ideal philosophy for a regulatory agency: "In all the areas of government regulation for which we are responsible, I think it is our obligation . . . to acquaint regulated people with what is required of them and to seek every possible inch of self-regulation, to ask for it, to try to get it.

"But failing to get it, I think it is our obligation to enforce this law vigorously, impartially, and impersonally, and to apply the sanctions of seizure, criminal prosecution, and injunction vigorously in those instances where voluntary compliance is not forthcoming with dispatch."[71]

If vigorous and even punitive actions are required, what protection does the regulated person or firm have? The FDA's decisions have rarely been reversed in the courts,[72] and for this reason drug sponsors do not resort to legal procedures so often as they might. Professor David Cavers of the Harvard Law School, writing in 1966, stated that: "In 27 years, under the 1938 and 1962 acts, about 13,000 applications [i.e., for approval of NDA's] have been processed and many denied or withdrawn. Yet only a single applicant has carried its case through the administrative hearing stage. Having lost there, it went no further." This was a hearing on the withdrawal of Altafur tablets, recommended for the treatment of infections caused by staphylococci.[73] Since then the Abbott Laboratories carried a case involving labeling to court and won it.[74]

Yet recourse to the courts is time-consuming and expensive. Can better protection be given to the rights of drug sponsors short of court procedure? The suggestion has been made that whenever the FDA decides to refuse or withdraw approval of a new drug, it be required to seek the advice of a committee of experts if the sponsor requests it.[75] Critics like Dean William C. Warren of the Columbia University Law School object to this procedure; they believe that the administrator in such a case has "abdicated his official function" because he fears that he will be criticized if he acts against the advice of the experts, whereas he expects to be shielded from criticism if he takes it.[76]

Yet, as I have pointed out before, the FDA cannot possibly have experts on its staff in every subject upon which it must rule. Also its position as simultaneous advocate and judge is often difficult. If it could find a fair and efficient method of utilizing outside experts before a decision was made on important issues, it could simplify its own work while giving the regulated industry assurance of the justice of its decisions.

Professor Cavers[77] recommends that the FDA follow the practices used by the Atomic Energy Commission in contested cases on safeguards for atomic energy reactors. Where neither the agency nor the applicant is ready to back down, the Atomic Energy Commission appoints a hearing board of two to four experts plus a lawyer as chairman.

One significant difference between the cases before the two regulatory agencies is their frequency. Nuclear reactors are not, at least at present, proliferating as rapidly as new drugs. If hearings were mandatory on request, it is possible that companies would always ask for them when a decision went against them, although this apparently has not happened in cases coming under the Pesticide Act, where appeal to an advisory committee is mandatory if requested by the sponsor.

I would suggest that when a crucial case involving a single sponsor or important cases involving a number of sponsors cannot be settled by negotiation, the FDA appoint a panel of experts under the chairmanship of a lawyer to hold a hearing at which the FDA and the sponsors would be present. The record of the hearing and the recommendations of the panel would be made public. These recommendations would not be binding upon the commissioner of Food and Drugs.

Originally much of the impetus for pure food and drug laws came from officials of state governments who were charged with enforcing local laws, were overwhelmed by the enormity of the task, and saw the need for control of products that crossed state lines, for more expertise, and for additional manpower, none of which the states could provide. While these individuals gave strong support to the passage of the food and drug acts in 1906 and 1938, the activities of state and city governments have languished in general.

All of the states have food and drug laws, but only thirty-four have laws that follow the Uniform Food, Drug and Cosmetic Act recommended by the Association of Food and Drug Officials of the United States. The FDA is working with

state officials to implement the passage and enforcement of
uniform laws. A good example is the passage in Illinois of a
strong food, drug, and cosmetic law in 1967. At the request of
that state the FDA lent one of its top executives to help plan
and set up the machinery to implement the new law.[78]

Clearly the FDA cannot do the whole job of surveillance
over drugs in the United States. First, it has no jurisdiction over
drugs produced and sold within a state. Second, it cannot keep
tabs on the hundreds of small establishments that produce drugs
mainly within a state, a few of which may be sold in neighbor-
ing states. Finally, a state government has a major interest in
retail stores, and in regulating these it may come upon facts that
are important to the federal regulatory program. On the other
hand, no state can expect to marshal the facilities and expertise
for the study and testing of drugs that the federal government
has, nor does it need to, since the federal experts and laboratories stand ready to give advice and help. It is to be hoped that
the state side of this partnership will be strengthened in the next
two decades as much as the federal portion has been improved
in the last two.

The trend in the regulation of drugs in this country has been
from private to governmental control, and from local control to
stronger and more comprehensive national control. In carrying
out the national commitment, are the federal regulatory agencies
hampered by their organization?

An independent commission for the regulation of drugs has
been recommended by some critics. But observation of presently
constituted commissions, such as the Interstate Commerce
Commission and the Federal Trade Commission, indicates that
independent status does not remove them from politics. Rather,
they have the disadvantage of being political units without the
advantage of more direct access to the power of the President,
which the Secretary of Health, Education and Welfare has as a
member of the Cabinet. Furthermore, one cannot be sure that
the independent commissions are freer from pressure by the

regulated industry than regulatory branches of Cabinet departments. A former commissioner of the Federal Communications
Commission confessed:

"It works subtly, almost silently like the water on a stone.
If you want to be reappointed you do not want to earn the
enmity of A.T. & T., a network, a multiple station owner. These
are really the insidious pressures."[79] An independent commission
does not seem to be the answer to the FDA's problems.

Whether the Division of Biologics Standards and the FDA
should be a single unit is another question. Theoretically, this
would be the ideal; if one were starting out today to structure
the regulation of drugs, including the biologicals, one would
probably place everything under one agency. Yet each agency
has now developed its *modus operandi* and its own *esprit*; there
is no point in risking the curtailment of their productivity by
tearing out the roots of tradition. The recent co-ordination of
all health affairs under an assistant secretary should serve to
bring the FDA and the Division of Biologics Standards closer
together. I have already discussed the establishment of a
separate unit at the National Institutes of Health for the study
of drugs and concluded that this divorce of the scientific from
the regulatory functions of the FDA would not be healthy.

If we assume that the present structure of these agencies
should not be tampered with, what recommendations can be
made for better regulation by the agencies as they stand? The
defects and inadequacies of the FDA and the Division of
Biologics Standards are mainly those of the federal government
in general and of regulatory agencies in particular. Morale of
the staff must arise from confidence in its professional excellence
and dedication to public service, rather than from a paranoid
delusion that the whole world is evil beyond the walls of the
agency. The leaders of the FDA must possess administrative
ability plus a high degree of excellence in a professional skill
basic to the activities of the agency, such as pharmacology,
pharmaceutical chemistry, microbiology, clinical medicine,
public health, or law. Administrators with various backgrounds
should be represented in the policy-making group. A free flow

of professionals from and to universities, research institutes, and the laboratories of the pharmaceutical companies is necessary, and for this and other reasons salaries must be competitive.

The Congress has as its duty the surveillance of the executive agencies, and painful though its whacks may be, it does sometimes serve to bring an agency forcefully into line with the public interest. But the multiplying of investigations of a single agency because the agency is at the time in the public eye, and thus an easy road to political notoriety, is hardly conducive to the building of a consistent policy of regulation or of high morale within an agency. Since 1958 the FDA has been investigated by seven committees, chaired by Congressman Blatnik, Senator Kefauver (two committees), Senator Humphrey, Congressman Fountain, and Senator Nelson. The problems of congressional hearings, such as the "trial by headline" and denial of the privilege of cross-examination, have been expounded by many others more competent than I. Until some reforms are made, the congressional committee will not be as effective an instrument for improving the federal regulatory agencies as it can be.

In concluding this chapter, a few words are in order on the interrelationships of private and public agencies concerned with drugs. Regarding the qualifications of investigators of new drugs, the role of the government should be to establish minimal criteria and to investigate cases where the data submitted suggest dishonesty or carelessness. The FDA is doing this now. The job of private groups should be to work out the qualifications of investigators for the different phases of clinical investigation. Whether the private groups will eventually develop a system of certification of investigators on the basis of training or examinations is a question that can be left for the future. Certainly we will not be ready for this for another decade at the least.

Coincident with the establishment of criteria, the private groups should work to elevate the standards of clinical investigators by providing more educational opportunities than are available at present, by disciplining members who do shoddy or dishonest work, and by rewarding those who do outstanding work. Discipline would be mostly at the local level in hospital staffs and in medical societies; awards should be at all levels.

The medical profession, the public, and the law have just begun to take cognizance of the problems involved in the consent of persons experimented upon. I believe that the public agencies should confine themselves to a general statement of principles and require sponsors to see that the responsibility of safeguarding the interests of the experimental subjects is assumed by proper professional groups, such as hospital committees. After sufficient experience is gained in hospitals, county medical societies should do the same for human investigations in doctors' offices. Admittedly, these would be harder to monitor, but once the word had spread among the profession and the public that the rules and the mechanism existed, I believe it could be done.

Once this machinery was working, the FDA should be requested to eliminate the regulations in which it spells out the circumstances under which consent and written consent should be obtained. In its place it could substitute a regulation requiring an institution or professional group to certify that it will be responsible for proper safeguards. Surveillance of the hospitals in turn would be carried out as a part of the periodic inspection of the Joint Commission for Accreditation of Hospitals. Local medical societies should be inspected by committees appointed by state or national societies.

I have stressed repeatedly the need for more information about how and why doctors use drugs as they do, and the therapeutic and adverse effects they obtain. Private and public groups alike should feel the responsibility for gathering this knowledge. As Alfred North Whitehead has said: "Where attainable knowledge could have changed the issue, ignorance has the guilt of vice."[80]

The public sector can do its part by awarding contracts and grants. In addition, the liaison between the FDA and the

262 *Medicines for Man*

262 Medicines for Man

National Institutes of Health should be improved so that the staffs and councils of the various institutes could be alerted to programs that would be of interest to the FDA. Some steps have already been taken in this direction.[81] More programs should be initiated within the institutes for the stimulation and awarding of grants for important areas of therapeutics. One method would be to place a representative of the FDA on the council of each institute, in addition to the representatives of the armed forces and the Veterans Administration, as at present.

The FDA probably has the largest corps of personnel and the greatest concentration of facilities in the world for the laboratory and animal testing of drugs. These are needed to regulate drugs in the nation that produces more drugs than any other, and to protect the interests of the public in the richest country in the world. These resources should be augmented and kept up to date. The facilities and personnel to evaluate efficacy, adverse effects, and biologic availability of drugs in humans should be brought up to the same level of competence. This would still leave much for private agencies to do. The FDA's evaluation of a drug should not be the sole evaluation. Rather, individuals and organized groups should make it their job to study drugs independently and voice their opinions consistently and firmly.

In addition, relative efficacy is beyond the purview of the FDA except where the vendors force the issue by claims of relative efficacy in their labeling or advertisements. It must be realized that regulation begets regulation. Regulation of labeling required the setting of standards; regulation of adverse reactions required consideration of efficacy. In the same way, regulation of efficacy is going to force inquiry into relative efficacy. But this need not be in the province of the public agencies. Just as the *USP* and *NF* took over the job of setting standards for most drugs, so relative efficacy can be determined by others and their findings accepted by the federal government, *provided* the job is done promptly and properly.

The final function of regulating agencies is the dissemination of information about drugs. If this is done properly it can do much to improve the practice of medicine and keep it at a high level.

Selecting generic names for drugs is an important factor in disseminating information. The machinery of the United States Adopted Names Council for naming new drugs is working well, but many older names are not so simple and as easily pronounced as they should be. I believe that the council should move rapidly to simplify these also. The FDA has rarely found it necessary to insist upon a name different from the one selected by the council. But its collaboration puts a club in the hands of the council that is effective even though seldom used. The partnership of interested groups in the naming of drugs is private-public collaboration at its best and should be emulated elsewhere.

With respect to advertising, I would recommend that as much as possible the actions of the FDA be limited to laying down general principles to be followed by drug firms and to spot-checking advertisements. Such general principles give editors of medical journals a code of minimum acceptability for advertisements and thus strengthen their hands when they need to reject those that are substandard. Journals of distinction will add their own rules, which may involve additional professional requirements and should certainly include standards of good taste. The FDA will thus be able to direct its attention to advertisements in journals whose editors will not assume their responsibility.

More important is the dissemination of information by other methods. In general, getting information to the drug manufacturers is no problem. In fact, reporters for trade journals are able to nose out the news of FDA actions even before it has reached all of the relevant personnel in the agency. A firm adherence to a carefully thought-out and consistently maintained philosophy is the best way to illuminate the road for the industry that must travel it. In this connection, these remarks written after the passage of the 1938 act are relevant:

> *It is improbable, moreover, that the Congress,*
> *despite its long wrangling over the provisions, grasped*

> *the full implications of the statute it finally enacted
> in 1938. Certainly it could not anticipate the impetus
> the law would give to drug therapy; and it is
> doubtful that it foresaw that compliance with the
> new requirements of the Act virtually compels the
> manufacturer and distributor of a drug . . . to apply
> the principles of rational therapeutics to his product
> if he is not, through inadvertency or otherwise, to find
> himself violating the law. The strict and unflinching
> enforcement policy that has characterized the
> activities of the Food and Drug Administration in
> carrying out its mandate under the statute has further
> implemented and directed the course of this
> development."*[82]

I am convinced that ten years from now, the 1962 law will be judged an even greater stimulus to the scientific and technological upgrading of the pharmaceutical industry. In spite of differences in some of their objectives, the FDA and the pharmaceutical industry have much in common, and those mutual interests will thrive by communication. As Bronowski has put it: "Science confronts the work of one man with that of another and grafts each on each; and it cannot survive without justice and honour and respect between man and man."[83]

But groups outside of industry must be reached better than in the past. Doctors, dentists, pharmacists, nurses, and other health professionals must become familiar with the mission of the FDA and how it affects them. Beyond this, regulatory agencies should be chary of disseminating scientific information and recommendations directly to the professions, because such a recommendation perforce takes on the character of a regulation and thus diminishes the scope of judgment so necessary to the best work of the professional.

On the other hand, the private groups need to improve considerably the transmission of information to professions on their part. This will be discussed in Chapter 13.

Finally, the public must be kept informed of the activities of the government regulatory agencies because in the end these agencies draw their support from the consumers of the country. The public must also be educated by private individuals and groups regarding the uses and adverse reactions of drugs, and, in emergencies, directly by the federal government.

There remain a sizeable number of regulatory functions for the public agencies; inspection of plants; testing samples of drugs; detecting and exposing quacks, incompetents, counterfeiters, and adulterators; and the prosecution of those who cannot, will not, or should not be brought into line by gentler measures. In all of these the agency needs expertise and financial and moral support. The regulated industry should co-operate where possible but has the right and duty to oppose by proper means those measures which it considers illegal, unduly restrictive, or not in the public interest. "The State is served poorly whether the bureaucracy dominates the interest group or the interest groups turn it to their own selfish ends. A proper working relationship must be established between the two."[84]

12

The Individual Doctor and Drug Therapy–Today

U p to this point we have been concerned mainly with the impact upon therapeutic advances of the laboratory scientist, the clinical investigator, and the administrator in government and industry. But as has been mentioned before, most drugs—and particularly all the highly effective ones, all those used in serious illnesses, and all those that are extremely toxic—must be prescribed by a physician. And what shall it profit a man if the drug he needs is discovered by a Nobel Prize winner, manufactured by the most up-to-date methods, inspected by the most conscientious of regulatory agencies, and sold at a low price, if his doctor doesn't know enough to give it to him when he needs it—or prescribes it improperly or in the wrong dose.

How much does the physician know about the drugs he prescribes? Where does he get his information? How good are his decisions about therapy? Can they be improved, and if so, how? As a background for these questions, let us first look at how the attitude of today's doctor toward therapeutics evolved.

We are not surprised to hear that at one time or another physicians believed in the efficacy of extracts and decoctions made from many of the common trees, weeds, and vegetables, such as hemlock, sassafras, May apple, pipsissewa, and rhubarb. We shudder to hear that the *Pharmacopeia Londonensis*, published in 1618, listed extracts made from ants, earthworms, grasshoppers, the eyes of crayfish, and the tails of lizards; powders from mummies; and the excrements of pigeons, mice, goats, and wolves.[1] We are appalled to learn that within a single year Louis XIII, who surely received the best medical care available in his day, swallowed at his doctor's direction 228 purges, was given 224 enemas, and was bled 42 times.[2]

This royal patient's experience serves to introduce the Age of Heroic Therapy, a period that was at its peak during the last quarter of the eighteenth century and the first quarter of the nineteenth. During this period patients were not only depleted by the removal of quarts of blood, sucked dry by leeches applied to the skin, and blistered with numerous irritants, but were also persuaded to swallow calomel and other mercury compounds in amounts that loosened the teeth as well as the bowels, along with countless powders, tinctures, and extracts. These ranged from bitter, foul, and nauseous to clean, sweet, and delectable— all the way from the pharmacologically worthless to the deadly poisonous. Worse still, in the rag bag of ineffective drugs the good ones sometimes got lost. The pharmacopeia of 1863 of the General Infirmary of Leeds contained no preparation of digitalis, even though Withering's thorough and well-documented study of its action on the heart and kidneys had been published in 1785.[3] Drugs were prescribed mostly from superficial impressions and personal prejudices. Doctors accumulated a set of favorite prescriptions that became their stock in trade and were collected as assiduously as some people gather *objets d'art.* Robert Boyle, the pioneer scientist of the seventeenth century, was less scientific in his approach to drugs than to the behavior of atmospheric gases. He prescribed mercury in beer for intestinal worms, recommended eating soap for bloody urine, and treated his own leg cramps by wearing a ring made from an elk's tooth.[4] The critical method, demanding that drugs be selected on rigid proof of their effectiveness, had not yet come to medicine.

Heroic therapy became less popular after the first quarter of the nineteenth century, but it still showed flutters of life. As late as 1878 Dr. H. C. Wood advocated bleeding patients with peritonitis until they fainted, then applying leeches to the abdomen, then dosing them with calomel, and finally knocking them out with huge doses of opium.[5]

Nevertheless, most doctors had seen the dangers, or at least the futility, of their ways and had begun to discard these heroic measures. But as in physics, so in physic, every reaction is followed by an equal and contrary reaction; the doctors, or at least their leaders, swung from over-therapy to therapeutic nihilism.

As early as 1846 John Forbes had concluded that since nature cured a high percentage of sick people and since some even recovered in spite of the injurious drugs the doctors gave them, therefore, "it would fare as well, or better, with patients, in the actual condition of the medical art, . . . if all remedies, at least all active remedies, especially drugs, were abandoned."[6] Tortuous prose, but containing a core of truth.

Much of this skepticism was justified, and healthy in its effects. Sir William Osler in the first edition of his famous text-book of medicine swept away many so-called remedies, hoary with age, in such phrases as: "no medicinal agents have any special or peculiar action upon tuberculous processes"; "[pneumonia] can neither be aborted nor cut short by any known means at our command," and, with respect to myxedema,* "unfortunately no satisfactory treatment is known."[7]

But the shift in attitude was often so extreme that therapy became the neglected stepchild of medicine, wasting in the shadow of her more favored sisters, Miss Brilliant Diagnosis and Miss Trustworthy Autopsy Examination. The critical faculty had come to the medical profession, but it was as yet poorly balanced.

Doctors trained in the school of therapeutic nihilism were ill prepared for the teeming harvest of the Age of Therapeutic Abundance. This period began toward the end of the nineteenth century and burst into full flower in the 1930's. By 1959 the number of new drugs introduced in a year was more than three hundred, plus an additional hundred new dosage-forms of already existing products. How did the practicing physician cope with the mass of information needed to use these large numbers of new drugs properly? So that the reader may draw his own conclusions, I shall cite some of the evidence. But first let us consider in detail how information about drugs reaches today's physician.

The *American Hospital Formulary Service*, published by the American Society of Hospital Pharmacists, lists about 3,000

---

* Myxedema is the disease in the adult which results from underactivity of the thyroid gland. Now that the cause is known, the patient is given a powder made from animal thyroid glands to substitute for what he cannot manufacture himself.

drugs. The *Physicians' Desk Reference,* which is sent free to all doctors, lists over 2,600 drug products. In 1967 over one billion prescriptions were filled in the United States, at a total expenditure of 3.3 billion dollars.[8] How much time is spent in learning about drugs by the doctors who write these prescriptions? In the second year of the four-year medical curriculum the student is introduced to the subject of drugs in his course in pharmacology. A survey published in 1954 revealed that this course occupied between 100 and 220 hours of the medical student's time in over two thirds of the nation's medical schools.[9] Only five of sixty-two schools reporting spent more than ten hours a week on this subject, including the lectures, seminars, and laboratory exercises—not much time for mastering a large and complicated subject.

As knowledge of the chemical structure of drugs has grown, and as scientists have learned more and more about the effects of drugs on individual cells, facts and concepts in these basic areas have occupied an ever increasing share of the attention of the teachers and a progressively larger part of the course in pharmacology. Their application has been left mainly to the third and fourth years of the medical curriculum, when the student works with patients on the hospital wards, in the outpatient clinics, and in the patients' homes. Here at last is the place for the student to learn to use drugs properly. But does he? Since it is important for the student to comprehend, first of all, the reason for the patient's disordered physiology, which we call disease, and to diagnose the patient's abnormality before anything else can be undertaken, the subject of treatment comes last and often receives little attention.

Also, instruction in the clinical years is provided by five large departments and a number of smaller ones. And there's the rub; the result may be confusion. There is little attempt at correlation, and when the venture is made it often founders on the rocks of individual beliefs based upon "personal experience." Sometimes it seems that we are no better off than we were nearly two centuries ago, as exemplified by an incident that occurred at that time at the University of Pennsylvania. When a student was criticized in an oral examination for speaking favorably of a quack medicine, Swain's Panacea, the professor of pharmacy, John Redman Coxe, pointed out that three of the leading professors in the medical school had written testimonials in praise of it.[10]

Thus, when students graduate from medical schools, their training in the use of drugs for the prevention and treatment of illness is spotty and often scanty. During the subsequent internship and residency training systematic study of drugs is rare, and though the recent graduate tries to plot a course of rational therapy based on the principles taught by pharmacologists, he tends to be blown off his route by the gusty gales of advertising and the cross winds of opinion among his colleagues. Such is his plight as he sails out of the protected harbor of internship and residency into the open seas of practice. How does he react to the sources of information available to him there?

Several surveys have been made in which physicians were asked where they obtained their first information about a drug or what source persuaded them to use it. These studies are open to several criticisms: the samples have not always been large enough nor the experiments properly designed so as to eliminate chance variation; the doctors may not always have recalled correctly the reasons for their actions or admitted to the real reasons; and finally, the way in which the questions were asked may have influenced the answers. Still, these studies provide the only information available, and they do give a rough idea of the various forces acting upon doctors. I shall refer to all of the published studies I have been able to find in which the data were adequate for tabulation.

Table 8 gives the results of three studies in which physicians were queried regarding their first information about a new drug. The detail man, who visits doctors' offices to push his company's products, was the source of the initial notice in 31 to 52 per cent of cases; medical journals in 9 to 25 per cent; and direct mail advertising in 16 to 22 per cent. If we assume that one fourth of the first notices from journals came from the advertising columns (and my own observations lead me to believe the figure should be much higher), it appears that

TABLE 8. Sources That Served as the First Notice to Doctors of the Availability of New Drugs

Source	*Per cent of doctors*		
	Caplow and Raymond study	*Ferber and Wales study*	*Coleman et al. study*
Detail men	31	38	52
Medical journals			
Articles	19	25	9
Advertisements	6		
Direct mail advertisements	16	19	22
Colleagues	14	6	10
Medical meetings	7	4	3
Other	7	8	3
Totals	100	100	99
No. of doctors			
answering	182	328	87

SOURCES: T. Caplow and J. J. Raymond, Jr.: "Factors Influencing the Selection of Pharmaceutical Products," *Marketing*, Vol. 19 (July 1954), pp. 18–23.
R. Ferber and H. G. Wales: "The Effectiveness of Pharmaceutical Promotion," *University of Illinois Bureau of Economics and Business Research Bulletin* 83, (Urbana, Illinois; 1958), p. 22.
J. S. Coleman, E. Katz, and H. Menzel: *Medical Innovation. A Diffusion Study* (Indianapolis: The Bobbs-Merrill Company, Inc.; 1966), p. 59.

from one half to three fourths of the time the first information about a new drug came from promotion by the drug company—whose interest it was to make the doctor use it.

Perhaps this is as it should be. Perhaps where the initial information comes from is not important. What about the sources that convince doctors to try drugs the first time? These are shown in Table 9. Here we see more disparity among the answers, which probably reflects the way in which the questions were phrased. In the survey by Coleman and his associates, 21 per cent of doctors were persuaded to prescribe the drug on the basis of direct promotion by a pharmaceutical company, and another 21 per cent because of what they read in a drug firm's periodical.[11] Ferber and Wales found that at least 39 per cent were induced to use a new drug by pressure from the seller,[12] while in the Gaffin study the corresponding figure was 67 per cent.[13]

TABLE 9. Sources That Led Doctors to First Use of a Drug

	Per cent of doctors		
Source	Coleman et al. study	Ferber and Wales study	Gaffin study
Detail men	5	21	41*
Medical journals			
Articles	42†	28	15
Advertisements	2		
Direct mail advertisements	14	18	26
Colleagues	28	13	7
Medical meetings	8	4	2
Other	1	16	9
Totals	100	100	100
No. of doctors answering	87	328	1,011

* Some doctors named more than one source. Percentages have been adjusted to 100 per cent.
† This includes professional journals (21 per cent) and periodicals published by drug companies (21 per cent).
SOURCES: J. S. Coleman, E. Katz, and H. Menzel: *Medical Innovation. A Diffusion Study* (Indianapolis: The Bobbs-Merrill Company, Inc.: 1966), p. 59.
R. Ferber and H. G. Wales: "The Effectiveness of Pharmaceutical Promotion," *University of Illinois Bureau of Economics and Business Research Bulletin* 83 (Urbana, Illinois; 1958), p. 24.
Attitudes of U.S. Physicians toward the American Pharmaceutical Industry (Chicago: Ben Gaffin and Associates, Inc.; 1959), p. C-13.

In the Gaffin survey, when doctors were asked which two or three sources they considered the most important for familiarizing themselves with new drugs, 68 per cent of doctors specified detail men, 32 per cent journal advertisements, 25 per cent direct mail advertisements, and 22 per cent drug samples.* This can be compared with 35 per cent who named medical meetings, 24 per cent who indicated conversations with colleagues, and 20 per cent who specified journal articles.[14] In a more recent survey, 62 per cent of physicians listed sources in the pharmaceutical industry among the first three sources of information they preferred, while only 35 per cent named medical journals or meetings and conversations with their colleagues as their choice of sources.[15] From the two surveys it appears that *doctors consider promotion by the company selling*

* The percentages add up to more than 100 because each doctor named more than one source.

the drug twice as important as information reaching them from their professional colleagues!

A British committee chaired by Lord Sainsbury investigated the reactions of 437 general practitioners to information about drugs. The doctors were given the names of four drugs that had recently been placed on the market and were asked whether they first prescribed the drug after hearing about it from a single source or from several sources. The percentage prescribing after learning about the drug from only one source varied from 31 per cent for indomethacin, a pain-relieving drug, to 61 per cent for fluocortolone, a variant in the long series of corticosteroid compounds that began with cortisone. Most amazing was the admission by the doctors queried that of those who prescribed a drug after hearing about it through one route, 9 per cent wrote the initial prescription after reading about the drug in advertisements and 39 per cent after being told about it by detail men.[16]

That the doctors were often captives of the drug firms' promotional methods was further shown by their responses to the question whether there was usually enough information in the literature promulgated by the drug firm to enable a general practitioner to decide whether or not to use a new drug. Among doctors below the age of thirty-nine, 27 per cent thought that there was enough information. This percentage increased progressively to 47 per cent for those fifty years of age or above.[17]

Finally, 46 per cent of general practitioners believed that they were able to decide whether to use a new drug solely on the basis of seeing a detail man.[18] It is interesting that this figure is almost the same as for the 47 per cent who thought that meetings held by drug firms were useful in getting to know about drugs and is not much different from the 60 per cent who thought that meetings organized by their own medical societies were useful for this purpose. Clearly, general practitioners in England also have great respect for—or a naive trust in—the promotional programs of drug companies.

If approximately half of the average doctor's decisions about drugs rest on the shifting sands of promotion, upon what does he rely for the other half? Coleman and his associates were particularly impressed with doctor-to-doctor contacts and how they influenced the use of a new drug. They found that some doctors began to use new drugs earlier than others. Such men were likely to be highly interested in medicine as a science and intimate socially with other doctors. The drug these authors investigated was introduced first through professional relationships among doctors and later through friendship ties; finally the relatively isolated physicians adopted it for a variety of reasons. These authors found that reading medical journals was an important source of information about a new drug but, surprisingly, that medical meetings were not.[19] In the other two studies shown in Table 9, medical colleagues and medical journals appeared to have had less impact. In the Gaffin study only about one fourth of the doctors were stimulated by a source within their profession to use a drug for the first time.

In view of the plethora of drugs on the market, the even larger number of brand names attached to them, the many different, and sometimes conflicting, sources of information, and the considerable dependence of the physican upon the promotion of drugs by the companies that sell them, how good is the doctor's selection? How well are the people of the United States being treated with drugs? The answer we must reluctantly give is "not nearly as well as they should be." What is the evidence for this harsh judgment?

Admittedly, evidence is hard to come by. In a highly individualistic profession, bred in the tradition of the frontier and placing a high premium upon independence, doctors have rebelled against being their brothers' keepers—so much so that they have at times allowed gross incompetence and charlatanism to flourish alongside the highest type of medical practice; yet a few studies have been made.

The quality of medical care may be measured by the outcome of the illness being treated. This criterion can best be applied in diseases that are invariably fatal unless proper treatment is given. For instance, some years ago my colleagues and I surveyed the records of all the patients with pneumococcic meningitis in the District of Columbia who had been treated with sulfa drugs, and classified them according to whether they received good, fair, or poor treatment. Ten per cent of those who had received good treatment survived; none of the others. Among those who died, the average survival time after diagnosis was 2.6, 2.1, and 1.2 days, for those who received good, fair, or poor treatment respectively.[20] (I might add that today much better results are obtained with penicillin therapy.) But such comparisons require sizeable numbers of patients in each group. And such clear-cut differences cannot be obtained in all diseases.

The number of reported deaths in the United States from what is called "therapeutic misadventure in the administration of drugs or biologicals" increased from 445 for the five-year period beginning in 1951 to 735 for the next five-year period, and to 890 for the five years beginning in 1961.[21] These figures certainly understate the actual number of deaths, because of failure to report some cases and because many deaths are classified under the organ or system affected by the drug. For instance, when a drug is used to treat congestive heart failure or to cure a disturbance in the rhythm of the heart, an adverse reaction would usually be classified under the cardiac abnormality for which treatment was given.

Since the criterion of outcome is of limited value in determining the quality of medical care, the criterion that is most used is the *process* of medical care. This requires setting standards for proper medical care, determined either by prevailing practice or by panels of experts or qualified practitioners.

In one study patients' hospital charts were reviewed by three internists, one of whom was a senior member of the hospital staff. Among 488 orders for individual drugs, 66, or 13 per cent, were considered to have been improper. In one case the dose was considered too high, in 17 too low, and in 3 cases another drug was judged to have been preferable. In 29 cases the diagnosis did not justify the use of any drug. Finally, in 16 cases, or 3 per cent of the total, the drug was considered to have been contraindicated; that is, its use would not only not help the patient but would probably do him harm.[22]

A survey of the use of antibiotics in seventy-six community

hospitals showed that 33.1 per cent of the patients were given antibiotics during January 1959, and 30.5 per cent in January 1961. But a search of over 85,000 patients' charts revealed a justifiable reason for the use of antibiotics in only 54 per cent of the patients who received them; over 39,000 patients in these hospitals received antibiotics unnecessarily during a single year.[23]

Another study also uncovered improper practices in the use of antibiotics. From the records of 1,490 operations for the repair of uncomplicated inguinal hernia performed in twenty-four hospitals in seven states, it was found that 38 per cent of the patients had been given antibacterial drugs. In 476 cases (84 per cent of those who received these drugs, or 32 per cent of all patients on whom this operation was performed), the antibiotics were given to prevent infection. But since infection should not occur following this operation if proper techniques are employed, these patients were subjected to needless risk and expense. Furthermore, when the entire group of 1,536 operations for both complicated and uncomplicated hernia were considered, the proportion of patients who received antibiotics varied from hospital to hospital all the way from 3 per cent to 82 per cent.[24] Clearly, if the doctors in the first hospital were right, those in the last were guilty of gross mismanagement, and vice versa.

Perhaps the most flagrant example of bad therapeutic judgment has been the failure of some doctors to desist from the unnecessary use of chloramphenicol. Within two years after this antibiotic was placed on the market, cases of aplastic anemia were reported. In 1952 a survey by the FDA of records of hospitals in the larger cities of this country revealed that among 539 persons with blood disorders, 143 persons had received chloramphenicol, along with one or more other drugs, and 55 persons had received cloramphenicol alone. More than half (53 per cent) of the patients with this disorder died.[25] I was a member of a committee convened by the National Research Council to consider the problem at the request of the commissioner of food and drugs. We recommended that chloramphenicol remain on the market, because it was necessary for the treatment of typhoid fever and certain other diseases, but that each package bear labeling warning doctors that its use had been associated with blood disorders. As a result of this and other publicity the sales of chloramphenicol fell sharply, but after 1954 they rose again, until in 1960 it was estimated that enough chloramphenicol was being sold to give a course of treatment with this antibiotic to more than 3.5 million persons.[26] Stronger warnings were required in the labeling early in 1961. Again the sales dropped, only to be followed by another rise. The new peak was essentially unaffected by minor changes in the labeling required in 1966, but as a result of the hearings of a committee chaired by Senator Nelson and the attendant publicity, accompanied by still more stringent labeling required in 1968 by the FDA, the quantity of chloramphenicol produced has fallen again—for how long, no one can say.[27]

Was the chloramphenicol used properly? Among 408 cases of blood disorders following the administration of chloramphenicol reported to the AMA, the disease for which it was given was specified in the case of 288 patients. In 12 per cent it was prescribed for the common cold (which is not affected by any antibiotic). In 15 per cent it was given for infections that would have responded better to another, less toxic antibiotic. In only 6 or 7 per cent of the cases was chloramphenicol the drug of choice, representing better therapy than other drugs that were less toxic.[28]

This is the way doctors used a dangerous drug, in spite of repeated warnings by experts, editorials in *The Journal of the American Medical Association* and other medical journals with wide distribution, stringent warnings on the labeling, and wide publicity in newspapers and magazines. Commissioner Goddard professed to be baffled by this method of practicing; Senator Nelson called it incredible.[29] How does one account for this apparent lack of knowledge on the part of so many doctors? It cannot be explained, except that the facts were obscured by a fog of advertising and by the smooth talk of detail men. Dr. Dickinson Richards claimed that: "The responsibility for using a new drug does reside finally in the practicing physician, and if he doesn't know about it, he simply hasn't done his homework."[30] Instead, doctors have been wheedled by winsome words, lured by loose allusion, fooled by fancy facts and figures, titillated by tantalizing testimonials, swamped in a sea of samples, and inveigled by itinerant influence men. The effect of such advertising has been that doctors often prescribe drugs by suggestion, rather than from a thoughtful evaluation of the facts.

Pressure to prescribe unwisely may come from patients also. I have been told frequently by practicing physicians that they give an antibiotic to a patient with a common cold, even though they know that it has no therapeutic effect, because the patient insists upon it and would go to another doctor, if necessary, to obtain it. One observer found that doctors occupy a spectrum all the way from those who are closely attuned to what their professional colleagues think and do to those on the other end who relate very little to their colleagues and are thus much more dependent upon their patients' attitudes and opinions. A physician in the latter group is less able to resist the importunities of his patients and therefore less likely to treat his patients on the basis of the best professional judgment.[31]

Granted that if a doctor falls behind the times, his patients might serve their own interests best by conveying the latest information from *Time* or *Newsweek*; yet the long history of errors perpetrated in the field of health by those without medical training makes the patient's uninformed judgment a poor substitute for the doctor's. This was shown in a study in which resident physicians were evaluated by their superiors, by their patients, by supervising nurses who worked on the same wards, and from the data that these physicians had entered on patients' charts. All the rankings correlated well except those made by the patients. The authors concluded that "patient happiness should not be accepted as *prima facie* evidence of patient welfare."[32]

The doctor's use of drugs also depends on how well he performs his other functions. A drug prescribed for the wrong disease is worse than no drug at all. Treatment rests squarely upon an understanding of disease processes, and a diagnosis, at least a tentative diagnosis, of the patient's illness is necessary before treatment is begun. Observations of thirty general practitioners in one city led to the conclusion that only five of them were "what their teachers in medical school wished them to be"; the other twenty-five made no serious attempt to establish a diagnosis, but prescribed on the basis of symptoms.[33] In other words, unlike the doctor in Matthew Arnold's poem who gave the ill he could not cure a name, these doctors gave the ill they could not name a drug.

These observations might be dismissed as one man's personal opinion if they had not since been substantiated by two thoroughly documented studies. The first consisted of observations of the work of eighty-eight general practitioners in North Carolina. Each doctor was rated on the various skills of general practice by an internist who watched him at work for three days, in the office, in the hospital, and in patients' homes. Therapeutic skills were assessed for six common disease categories. Proper treatment was judged to have been given for anemias by only 15 per cent of doctors, for emotional problems by 17 per cent, for congestive heart failure by 25 per cent, for upper respiratory infections or obesity by 33 per cent, and for hypertension by 43 per cent.

Although at first glance these judgments might seem too severe, the examples of faulty practice that were cited would be considered substandard by any good physician. Some of these were: giving penicillin for the common cold; treating anemia by "shot-gun" preparations that were claimed to have a therapeutic action in many varieties of anemia but actually were effective in few or none; prescribing an assortment of drugs for nonexistent organic disease in patients whose problems were emotional; shifting from drug to drug in treating high blood pressure, rather than adjusting the dose of a drug, or the intervals between doses, before deciding the drug was ineffective; and finally in heart failure an inexact or completely unscientific use of digitalis—a drug that has been thoroughly studied and the properties and uses of which have been carefully taught to the last two generations of medical students.

The observers found that doctors who practiced good therapy were likely to excel in other areas: diagnosis, prenatal and child care, as well as surgery and obstetrics. They concluded: "There was a remarkable consistency in the performance of the individual physician. That is to say, if he scored high on history-taking his performance in the other categories tended to be of the same order. If he did not perform a careful examination, it was unlikely that he would obtain a good history or prescribe rational treatment."[34]

The same method was used to survey the practices of forty-three general practitioners in Ontario and forty-two in Nova Scotia. Ratings were made by a pediatrician, an internist, and a specialist in public health. The findings were distressingly similar to those of the first study. When therapy was assessed in five different categories of diseases—infections, anemia, cardiac failure, hypertension, and obesity—the proportion of Ontario physicians whose work was considered unsatisfactory varied from 15 per cent for the treatment of cardiac failure to 75 per cent for the treatment of high blood pressure. Corresponding figures for Nova Scotia physicians ranged from 45 per cent for drugs used to treat infections to 75 per cent for high blood pressure.

Again, some of the actions of individual physicians were even more damning than the over-all ratings might imply. One doctor "handed a patient a box containing 1-milligram, 2-milligram, and 4-milligram tablets [of Corticosteroids], but gave neither instructions about dosage nor any warning about manifestations of overdosage."[35] (These powerful drugs have an action like that of the hormone from the cortex of the adrenal gland. Overdosage may cause high blood pressure, a diabetes-like condition, obesity, changes in the skin, ulcers of the stomach and intestines, fractures of bones, and psychoses.)

What can we conclude from these revelations? Are doctors practicing abysmally poor medicine, including therapeutics? Does the patient take his life in his hands every time he consults a physician, even for a minor ailment? Or have the faults of a small fraction been attributed to the medical profession as a whole? Are we dealing only with the minimum of error that cannot be eliminated because all humans err sometimes?

It is true that an investigation of the performance of any professional group would reveal a spectrum extending all the way from those whose work was excellent to those who were careless, lazy, ignorant, or just plain stupid. Then, too, some doctors complain that the academicians making the assessments are like the officials in a track meet who start the bar so high that only a few of the jumpers can qualify. Yet we must expect more of doctors than of any other calling. Compared with other professions, their training is the longest; they are more highly selected than most; and their actions affect the health, happiness, and life of everyone at one time or another. Under the circumstances, the number of doctors whose performance does not meet reasonable criteria of quality is too great to be tolerated. Unless we can improve the situation, we will have to admit that Matthew Prior's lament, written over two centuries ago, is still true today:

> *Cur'd yesterday of my disease,*
> *I died last night of my physician.*

Because I believe that improvement is possible, I shall consider in the next chapter the measures available for improving the quality of medical care, particularly drug therapy, and how they can be employed to change conditions for the better.

> ... the family doctor, the private in our great
> army, the essential factor in the battle, should
> be carefully nurtured by the schools and carefully
> guarded by the public. . . . No class of men
> needs to call to mind more often the wise
> comment of Plato that education is a life-long
> business.
>
> —SIR WILLIAM OSLER

> This is my vow: To perfect my medical art and
> never to swerve from it so long as God grants me
> my office, and to oppose all false medicine and
> teachings. . . . Not to judge anything superficially,
> but by symptoms, not to administer any medicine
> without understanding. . . . Not to guess but
> to know.
>
> —PARACELSUS (1493–1541)

13

The Individual
Doctor and Drug
Therapy—Tomorrow

In the last chapter we found that therapy with drugs is not all it should be. In this chapter I shall consider the methods used at present to inform, persuade, stimulate, or otherwise influence the physician so that he uses drugs to their best advantage, and how these methods can be improved.

One thing is certain: drugs cannot be prescribed by decree from a central authority. In the middle of the Civil War the surgeon general of the army, William Hammond, asserting that calomel had been used in excessive doses and that milder measures had failed to correct the abuse, ordered it removed from the list of drugs from which medical officers could prescribe. Although time has proved him right, that patients are better off without this highly toxic mercury compound, the medical practitioners of that day were not ready for a change. A storm of protest rose from doctors within and without the army. The editor of the *Philadelphia Medical and Surgical Reporter* was one of the more temperate critics. His suggestion was "why not throw out the ignorant men rather than the drugs?"[1] But Hammond was thrown out instead.

Is this not a lesson to those who would have the FDA set itself up as the arbiter of drug therapy? This agency is directed to prevent sponsors from giving doctors incorrect information about drugs and to supply doctors with the true facts if such an action is necessary to correct misinformation. Thus the FDA declares certain areas off limits; the doctor enters them at his own peril—at the risk of harming his patient or of being sued for malpractice. Within the wide territory that remains, the FDA is not directly concerned with how the doctors treats his patients.

The pharmaceutical industry also has a broad national impact upon the practice of medicine. Improvements in advertising resulting from new laws and regulations will materially assist the practicing physician. For even when the doctor has ready access to correct information on a particular drug, an improper advertisement can be distracting, making it hard for the doctor to correlate and utilize the information available. Elsewhere I have compared the advertising of drugs to driving an automobile on a city street at night.[2] Drivers learn to ignore the multicolored lights as they flicker on and off and to concentrate on the signal lights instead. But even the good driver is distracted by lights that are too bright, too glaring, too close to the signal lights, or too like them in color. So the best of doctors is sometimes distracted and even deluded by blatantly false or insidiously misleading advertising of drugs.

Since neither the federal government nor the drug industry should be the principal source of the doctor's information on drugs, what should these sources be? Let us first look at the information the doctor needs. It includes first, basic information on the composition and action of drugs; second, new information on old or new drugs that does not have to reach the doctor in a hurry; and third, information about old or new drugs that must be disseminated immediately, as soon as it becomes known.

Basic information is supplied mostly by medical scientists in medical schools and research institutes, and to a lesser extent by those in industry.

New information about old drugs is constantly being uncovered. It may reveal a new use for an old drug. For instance, quinine, the stand-by against malaria for centuries, was shown many years ago to correct certain disturbances in cardiac rhythm. On the basis of these findings an analogue was developed, quinidine, which was much more effective for this purpose and is in common use today.

More often, the new information consists of disproving the supposed effectiveness of a drug. In his presidential address before the Association of American Physicians in 1939, Dr. Eugene DuBois condemned the system by which a "huge number of useless drugs . . . are carried along from year to year in our teaching and practice." He likened such drugs to barnacles on the bottom of a boat and suggested that his audience, composed mostly of teachers in medical schools, had a duty to scrape them off at frequent intervals. "Any young neophyte can introduce a new drug," he added. "It requires a man of large experience and considerable reputation to destroy an old one."[3]

Although information about new drugs needs to be supplied to practicing physicians at a reasonable time after it becomes known, for many drugs this is not urgent. The physician may not have occasion to use the new drug for months or years. Or when he does need a drug of this class, an established drug that is just as good is often available. Moreover, the physician is handicapped if he hears of a new drug or a new use for an existing one without at the same time learning something about its mode of action and other important details. Accordingly, wherever the incorporation of new knowledge into the doctor's fund of information is not urgent, it is best that it come to him with other facts that will help him assimilate it and retain it properly.

On the other hand, some new drugs represent a radical departure from previous therapy, a lifesaving or symptom-allaying remedy where no drug was available before or previous ones were definitely inferior. Such were sulfapyridine for pneumonia, streptomycin for tuberculosis, penicillin for a host of infections, diphenylhydantoin for epilepsy, and *Rauwolfia* for high blood pressure. It has been my observation that most doctors quickly become aware of the existence of such drugs. They are abundantly publicized in the medical press, in medical meetings, and by word of mouth among physicians—and they are adopted promptly. Real coin of the realm always rings true.

Although Bernhard Stern, a noted sociologist, has drawn attention to the failure of the medical profession in the past to accept certain new concepts of disease or utilize effective new remedies,[4] I have found the opposite to be true in modern therapeutic practice. Today's physician is used to the sudden appearance of drugs that are more efficacious or less toxic than those he has at hand. And this creates a problem. A doctor may hear of a new drug that lowers blood pressure, stops the pain of gout, checks infections of the bladder caused by bacteria that were unaffected by any previous therapy, or enables an infertile woman to become pregnant. What he may not know is under what conditions the drug will work, how best to measure its results, when to stop treatment, and above all, what adverse reactions to look for.

In contrast to the readiness with which doctors sometimes begin to use a new drug, they do not always seem to be aware of adverse reactions that call for caution in the use of certain older drugs. Perhaps this is because adverse reactions are often not detected until a drug has been used many times; perhaps because doctors are not so willing to talk about poor results as about good ones; perhaps because advertising in the past has not stressed adverse reactions and has even played them down; or perhaps because doctors as well as other people get in a rut and the rut is sometimes deep. Whatever the reason, we need to devise better methods of alerting doctors about hazardous reactions from drugs and of stressing the risks attendant on their use.

Keeping up with the published information on adverse reactions is a Herculean task. Over a thousand journals published throughout the world devote at least half of their pages to research in toxicology.[5] Some reports of adverse reactions may be published in relatively obscure journals, even though the widely read journals try to stress such reports. *The Journal of the American Medical Association*, in particular, pays much attention to this field, because of the continuous interest of the Council on Drugs and because the editors have always recognized the responsibility of the journal with the largest circulation to keep physicians informed on this important subject.[6]

Because no one journal or group of journals can keep up with the pace of new knowledge, a number of abstracting and indexing services have sprung up. There is, of course, a considerable time lag between the publication of an article and its incorporation into an index or volume of abstracts. More and more the computer is being called upon to bridge the gap. The most extensive service is MEDLARS of the National Library of Medicine. Information is stored on magnetic tape, and searches are made on individual topics upon request. Several private services are also in operation. Some hospitals are trying experiments in which information about drugs is stored on a computer and made available to physicians right on the wards. It has been suggested that a national network should be devised to allow immediate access to information stored on a central computer connected to computers in individual hospitals. Meanwhile, physicians can obtain immediate information on a suspected adverse reaction or the therapeutic effect of a drug in a specific condition by telephoning the manufacturer, the Department of Drugs of the AMA, or the FDA.

Many of the practicing physician's needs do not involve new information and therefore may be met by standard textbooks of medicine or therapeutics. Yet these do not always go into sufficient detail to answer a specific question, nor do they include all drugs. It is a strange by-product of our Alice-in-Wonderland, federal-state system that no complete list of the drugs sold in this country exists, not even at the FDA, since drugs may be produced and sold within some states without the inspection, regulation, or even knowledge of any state authority, and federal laws have not been applied to intrastate drugs.

The book most widely used by the practicing physician, the *Physicians' Desk Reference*, is distributed free because each listing is actually a paid advertisement. In the past it could not be depended upon for unbiased information; since the FDA has been regulating the advertising of drugs, many of the statements have been drastically changed. But this book is not an authoritative source of information. Because of the source of its revenue it cannot make statements on the comparative efficacy or relative toxicity of drugs. Also, drugs sold by sponsors who are unwilling to pay do not get into the book.

Large loose-leaf indexes are available that list the properties and effects of the important or widely sold drugs. An example is the American Hospital Formulary Service. Since these are cumbersome and expensive, they are usually found only in libraries and the pharmacies of larger hospitals. Furthermore, they do not compare drugs nor make authoritative evaluations.

The pressure for a drug compendium listing all the drugs for sale in the United States and giving authoritative information about them has been mentioned previously. In Chapter 11 I recommended that nongovernmental, professional groups try to fill this need.

The deficiencies in the teaching of therapeutics in the medical schools of this country were discussed in Chapter 12. Some attempts at improvement have been made. One hope lies in the pharmacology and therapeutics committees of hospitals used for teaching medical students. By requiring clinical teachers to look closely at what drugs they are giving to patients, these committees force them to examine what they are teaching students. They will be discussed further when the use of drugs in hospitals is considered.

An important movement is the development of clinical pharmacology units in medical schools. These units have a triple purpose—teaching, research, and service—some units accentuating one and others another.[7] The need for research on the actions of drugs in humans and the mechanisms responsible for these actions has been stressed in previous chapters, as has the need for more teams of experts to evaluate new drugs as they appear. We are here concerned with the teaching function.

One aim of clinical pharmacology units is to produce more investigators who are competent to study drugs in humans. This will affect the medical student only if many of these experts, after they are trained, become teachers in medical schools. The other educational contribution of these units is to weld into a comprehensive whole the bits of information that the medical students receive elsewhere and to show them how to detect and discard the spurious ones. Since the task is huge and since clinical pharmacology units thus far have had small staffs, they have acted mostly to inform and stimulate the rest of the faculty. This may be enough, but to be effective these units need the strong support of the heads of the larger clinical departments as well as of the department of pharmacology and of the administration. They also need more financial help from the drug industry or the federal government.

Although no other comprehensive plan has been proposed, several interesting experiments in teaching have been tried. In one medical school, students read advertisements about drugs, followed by articles about the same drugs in medical journals. In class they reported on the compatability (or incompatability) of the two sources of information, following which the instructor added his opinions. It was found that the juxtaposition of advertisements and scientific articles stimulated the students to think carefully about the validity of the claims made for the drugs and to reach conclusions which corresponded closely with those of the faculty.[8]

At the University of Pennsylvania students participated in a double-blind evaluation of drugs in patients with anxiety or depression. At the end of the twelve-week period the code was broken and the results of the drug or placebo medication were revealed. The students learned not only the effects of the particular drugs studied, but also how a study is designed and carried out and how to judge the effects of drugs in general.[9]

At the University of Florida the pharmacology course has been split, the basic portion being taught in the second year and the clinical part in the fourth year, after the student has had his clinical experience. The students have shown more enthusiasm for the subject than formerly, and this has been reflected in a rise in the scores for pharmacology in nation-wide examinations.[10] These experiments show that when teachers are interested, progress can be made. The tragedy is that so few have been incited to action.

The solution cannot be the addition of more time to teach therapeutics. The curriculum of the medical school is already too crowded. Those interested in heart disease, cancer, mental disease, rheumatism, the economics of medical care, and a host of other subjects all demand more time in the medical curriculum. Each pressure group wants a bigger spot in the curricular sun. Meanwhile, the liberals on the faculty press for fewer required subjects and more electives, and the public is asking why the four-year period cannot be shortened.

The solution is not more time, but more correlation of the scattered hours and minutes now being spent in studying about drugs and watching their effects in patients. While agreeing that teaching and research in the laboratory and in animals must continue, I believe that from the beginning of the pharmacology course, teaching must be related as much as possible to the actions of drugs on people. Finally, I suggest that in some way we must obtain closer agreement among the faculty on the value of particular drugs. Granted that complete unanimity on scientific matters is neither possible nor desirable, yet when the members of a major department insist upon the wholesale use of chloramphenicol after repeatedly hearing members of other clinical departments cite the reasons why it should be used with caution, something is wrong. I would recommend that the fundamental knowledge of the pharmacologists, the therapeutic expertise of the clinicians, the feedback from surveys of the use of drugs in the hospitals used for teaching, should all be correlated in seminars in the senior year of medical school. By presenting and defending their viewpoints, faculty members would learn the newer basic concepts and practical applications along with the students.

In this country, the first year after graduation from medical school is almost invariably spent in an internship, and most doctors take further training as residents in one of the specialty areas or in general practice. As a house officer the young doctor is plunged into the middle of therapeutics. He is prescribing drugs for, and administering drugs to, dozens of patients in the hospital and in the outpatient service. During his first weeks as an intern his decisions on therapy will be supervised closely in hospitals that stress teaching. In other hospitals, the supervision will vary from patient to patient, depending upon the knowledge of the patient's attending physician and his interest in teaching. In the resident years many of the decisions on therapy are made by the resident himself. In puzzling or difficult cases, when new drugs are being used, or when catastrophes occur that might have been related to therapy, discussions on drugs often take place. They are sometimes informative, sometimes sketchy, sometimes thought-provoking, and sometimes merely a rehash of what can be found in a standard textbook. Seldom is any systematic attempt made by the hospital staff to make sure that the neophyte learns to practice rational therapy.

Also, for the first time the intern and resident physician are exposed to the blandishments of the detail man. In many hospitals he has the run of the wards, where he may be seen at any hour doling out samples to house officers and even to nurses. For he knows that if he can get a doctor to use a drug once, the doctor is likely to use it again, and if he can get the drug's trade name imprinted in the mind of the novice, that drug may be prescribed for years to come.

Gleaning their knowledge from varied sources, assimilating it while they try to learn a host of new skills, and utilizing it amid the stress of caring for desperately ill patients, many house officers find that while the sum of what they have learned about drugs may be large, the facts are always scattered, often ill-assorted, and sometimes discordant. More important, they realize that their understanding of how drugs work is slipping away. Some verification of this was obtained in the study of general practice in North Carolina; there was no correlation between length of a doctor's hospital training and the quality of therapy he practiced.[11]

Equipped with many facts about drugs but with a meager understanding of how to evaluate them and how best to select them, the young doctor plunges into the problems of practice. The average doctor will practice medicine for forty-five years after graduation. Where will he get his information about drugs, and how will he increase his understanding? He may take postgraduate courses, go to medical meetings, and attend conferences at hospitals. Among ninety-three general practitioners in North Carolina, thirty were given credit by the Academy of General Practice for less than 20 hours of postgraduate study during the preceding year, while only fifteen were credited with 60 hours or more. Attendance at medical society and hospital staff meetings increased as the hours of credit rose.

As might be expected, the quality of practice was lowest among doctors with the smallest amount of postgraduate study and rose with increase in postgraduate study up to 40 to 59 hours per year. Above this it fell somewhat. Is this because 50 hours per year is the most that can be properly integrated into a busy rural general practice, or because those who pursued postgraduate study most vigorously were unhappy in their daily work and unconsciously seeking an escape?[12]

Whatever the optimal time that should be allotted to postgraduate courses, my observation while teaching in these courses has been that the physicians who attend are usually interested, alert, eager to learn, and already know something about the subject, as judged by their questions. Many times we teachers have asked ourselves, "Wouldn't these men find a way to learn, whether they came to these courses or not?"

On the contrary, this does not seem to hold for medical society meetings. While some doctors in attendance listen attentively, take notes, ask questions, and are obviously there to learn, others apparently attend for social reasons, because it is a good means of "getting away," or because they are interested in the political affairs of the medical society. Perhaps this is why so few doctors credit medical meetings with contributing to their knowledge about drugs. (See Tables 8 and 9.)

What has been said refers to postgraduate education in general and not to therapeutics alone; the teaching of therapeutics cannot be improved without reforming the whole. It seems to me that in postgraduate medical education we are about where we were in undergraduate medical education in the 1890's. Short, unconnected courses, repeated year after year, seldom graduated from elementary to advanced, but given almost at random and irrespective of the student's previous education—these were characteristic of undergraduate education seventy-five years ago and are seen in postgraduate education today.

But change is in the air. Medical schools, hospitals, medical societies, and practicing physicians—all are becoming more interested in continuing medical education. In the school year 1966–1967 over 164,000 physicians registered for postgraduate courses. They chose from among nearly three thousand courses, which lasted from one day to several weeks, given by medical schools, hospitals, medical societies, and other groups. Medical schools alone enrolled 19,000 doctors in postgraduate courses in the school year 1954–1955, and nearly 140,000 in 1967–1968.[13]

Except for the introduction of television and other newer
visual aids and a few experiments in programmed instruction,
the courses have followed traditional patterns. Only an occasional
course among those listed by *The Journal of the American
Medical Association* is labeled "advanced."[14] Thus, graded courses
are practically nonexistent, unless one counts the 27 per cent of
the courses that are restricted to specialists. Directors of courses
have rarely tried to find out what the doctor knows before he
enters, and only occasionally do they give an examination when
the course is over. To me these procedures seem to be a *sine qua
non*. It is axiomatic that to teach properly we must take off from
the present level of a student's knowledge. At present, doctors
learn by word of mouth, or by trying for themselves, whether a
particular course fits their needs. But such a system wastes the
time of student and teacher.

The American College of Physicians has devised an examination for internists that can be taken by the doctor himself. Only
the examinee knows the results; he can use them to learn where
his deficiencies lie. Such a test could be devised for applicants
for each postgraduate course. The results, while kept confidential,
could be used to classify the applicants according to their fund
of knowledge and ability to apply it. Courses could then be set
up at different levels, planned explicitly to supply the deficiencies
uncovered by the tests.

At the end of a course the simplest way to test its effectiveness is to examine the information, skills, and attitudes of the
students. The simplest, but not the best. Such examinations should
be given; they can measure whether the doctor-student is ready
to move on to a more advanced course. But in postgraduate
education, unlike the undergraduate variety, the true test lies
close at hand: the doctor will be applying immediately what he
has learned. We should find out how well he does this. Obviously
we cannot monitor every doctor or every course in this way.
But selected courses can be carefully studied by observing the
doctors in their practices, with their consent, before and after the
course. Less time-consuming surveys can be made by asking
physicians, in interviews or in questionnaires, what changes they

have made in their methods of practice following a postgraduate course.[15] Studies such as these should tell us what kinds of postgraduate instruction are achieving our purpose—to improve the practice of medicine by physicians, with the eventual goal of giving people better health care.

In a survey of postgraduate education in the United States it was estimated that 30 to 50 per cent of doctors never undertake postgraduate work of any kind.[16] In a study of postgraduate education in Utah, in which 426 practicing physicians answered questionnaires, the primary obstacle to continuing education seemed to be that the doctors were too busy. " 'Too many patients' was the complaint of 37 per cent of the entire group and of 51 per cent of the general practitioners."[17]

What can be done to overcome the obstacle of insufficient time? This is especially important in a period when the chronic shortage of doctors will continue for a least another ten years before increasing enrollments in medical schools can possibly catch up with the demand. More group practice, more centering of medical practice around hospitals, and the training of assistants who can take over some of the services that doctors now perform —all will help.

The doctor can learn much in his own office. He should subscribe to and read several medical journals and the *Medical Letter*, which brings up-to-the-minute information and expert opinion on drugs. In addition to standard textbooks he should own *New Drugs* and *AMA Drug Evaluations* (when it is published). He should maintain a file of the latest information on drugs, consisting of brochures published by sponsors, package inserts, and warning letters issued by drug companies or the FDA.

Making the doctor's own hospital a center of education is an important way of saving his time by bringing new knowledge directly to him. A number of medical schools have developed continuing education programs in conjunction with hospitals some distance away. A further step, and an important one, is to develop a faculty for postgraduate instruction from the hospital's own staff. Thus the hospital becomes a viable teaching center, capable of planning and action on its own, and the medical school can divert its resources to some other institution that is asking for its help.

Television and programmed instruction are being tried as methods of bringing postgraduate study to the doctor. But in my opinion, we should not adopt them widely without finding out how much the doctor uses them and what impact they have on doctors' practices. This can best be done by studying one or two programs thoroughly, rather than by following the will-o'-the-wisp of gadgetry under the delusion that it must be worthwhile because it is being talked about so much.

Standards for hospitals throughout the United States are set by the Joint Commission on Accreditation of Hospitals, a voluntary group composed of representatives of the American College of Physicians, American College of Surgeons, American Hospital Association, and American Medical Association. The medical staff in an approved hospital is charged with the "surveillance of patient care provided in the hospital." Responsibility for proper drug therapy is usually divided among several committees. The Records Committee insures that the medical records describe "the therapy provided, the results thereof, and the placement of responsibility for all actions taken. . . ." The Medical Audit Committee reviews records to see whether proper medical care has been given. The Utilization Review Committee evaluates "the services ordered and provided . . . ," chiefly with respect to whether they have affected the length of stay of the patient in the hospital. Finally, the Pharmacy and Therapeutics Committee surveys the "pharmacy and therapeutic policies and practices . . . to assure optimal utilization with a minimum of potential for hazard."[18]

Since inspections are made by the joint commission at infrequent intervals and since hospitals vary greatly in size and quality of staff, the diligence with which these tasks are performed differs greatly from hospital to hospital. Furthermore, in 1967, among the 7,253 hospitals in the United States, only 1,700 hospitals were accredited—usually the larger ones.[19]

The Pharmacy and Therapeutics Committee may meet only once a year, and may have so little influence that the doctors prescribe whatever they wish. At the other extreme, this committee may establish a closed formulary, a list of drugs from which the doctor must prescribe. This is unusual. A larger number of hospital committees establish formularies containing the drugs they consider adequate for patient care and including those preparations and brands that come up to the highest standards but at the same time can be purchased at a reasonable price.

Burkholder found that among forty-five major teaching hospitals that replied to a questionnaire, six had committees that were not active. Of the remainder, twenty-three had developed their own formularies, which contained from 292 to 696 items.[20] Generally in smaller hospitals and in nonteaching hospitals these committees tend to be less active.

Hospital formularies have become more important since the enactment of the Social Security Amendments of 1965, which state that the cost of drugs given to hospitalized patients will be reimbursed under the Medicare program only if the drug is listed in certain national compendia or in a formulary adopted by the pharmacy and therapeutics committee of the hospital.

. What is the relationship of the individual doctor to the hospital formulary? A survey of general hospitals in New York City revealed that 89 per cent of 104 responding hospitals had a formulary and 7 per cent were developing one. One third of the hospitals required that prescriptions be limited to preparations in the formulary. These were usually public or large private hospitals. When a nonformulary drug was desired, it could be obtained simply on the doctor's request in 24 per cent of hospitals, while 40 per cent required the approval of the chief of the service, the pharmacy and therapeutics committee, or the administrator of the hospital.[21]

Formularies have become an explosive issue—not because anyone opposes the listing of drugs or the recommending of certain ones, but because prices of different preparations of the same drug sometimes vary so much that money can be saved if prescriptions can be restricted to cheaper preparations. If a committee composed of qualified physicians and a pharmacist selects the preparations and limits its choices to brands proved satisfactory by testing, by previous use, or by the reputation of the manufacturer, the patient will receive the best therapy available at the lowest cost to the purchaser.

Data on the physiologic availability of different brands of certain drugs have been published, and information is being obtained for other drugs. When the various brands of a drug have not been tested for therapeutic effects in patients and the physiologic availability of the various brands has not been determined, pharmacy and therapeutics committees are well advised to purchase a brand made by a company with a reputation for reliable products. There is nothing to prevent obtaining bids from several such companies, however, and purchasing from the lowest bidder.

When a physician insists that the brand he prefers be prescribed even though it is not in the formulary, some hospitals allow this without question. If the opinions of experts on the pharmacy and therapeutics committee and the information that comes to the pharmacists about preparations are of any value— and I think they are—they should not be so lightly swept aside. A few hospitals take the opposite tack and refuse to dispense anything that is not on the approved list. Although this is a reasonable policy for certain large hospitals in which members of the staff are carrying on research on drugs and thus have unusual knowledge in the area of therapeutics, for most hospitals it seems wise to allow some leeway to the prescribing physician. One simple way to do this is to dispense the nonformulary drug on his request the first time it is asked for, but not a second time, unless he has, in the meantime, presented to the pharmacy and therapeutics committee good reasons why this drug should be stocked in the pharmacy. Another method is to require the permission of the chief of the service or of the medical director of the hospital.

Another hotly debated question is whether the pharmacist should substitute a brand of a drug for the brand the doctor has prescribed. This practice is illegal in some states, and rightly so, in my opinion, because the final decision should remain with the prescriber, who has the ultimate responsibility. But surely there is nothing wrong with a medical staff's deciding that it will delegate to the Pharmacy and Therapeutics Committee the responsibility for selecting a suitable brand. This can be done by having each physician give written consent beforehand for the pharmacist to substitute the brand of any drug that has been approved by the proper authority. Such a procedure prevents wasteful duplication of several brands of the same drug on the pharmacy shelves, and allows for competitive bidding and group purchases, thus lowering the cost to the hospital and ultimately the price paid by the consumer.

To return to the effect of pharmacy and therapeutics committees and formularies upon the doctor's practice, it is evident that they can influence the doctor through education and by regulation. When a physician finds that the drug he has been using is not in the approved formulary, he should discuss the matter with a member of the committee or a pharmacist. In the conversation, or from the literature to which he will be referred, he may learn that the drug has been omitted because of adverse reactions with which he was not familiar or that it has been superseded by a more effective drug.

In the case of the occasional physician who insists upon prescribing drugs that have been proved to be inferior to other drugs, tough-minded pharmacy and therapeutics committees have a coercive effect. They place on medical practice a floor below which the doctor cannot go. As a profession, doctors must face the fact that such coercion is necessary at times if adequate standards are to be upheld.

Dr. Margaret McCarron, chairman of the Therapeutics Committee of the Los Angeles County General Hospital, summarized the value of a good hospital formulary system in testimony before a Senate committee:

> . . . the drug formulary system at the Los Angeles County General Hospital provides the staff with standard, familiar medications and enough information to use the drugs intelligently. It has improved the teaching of physicians and nurses and thus affords an added degree of protection for the patients.
> It has eliminated from the drug supply at the

> *hospital those items with little or no therapeutic*
> *effectiveness, has substituted some toxic agents with*
> *less toxic ones, has replaced some very expensive*
> *items with less costly ones, and has allowed the*
> *pharmacy to maintain a manageable inventory.*[22]

All of the surveillance of drug therapy in the hospital cannot be left to the Pharmacy and Therapeutics Committee. It has little to do with what happens after the doctor prescribes a drug, although its records are of value in tracing adverse reactions and making studies of effectiveness. The committees that must determine whether the proper drug was prescribed, in the proper dosage, and for the proper period of time, are the Medical Audit and the Utilization Committees. As these committees become more active in hospitals, and as doctors become used to the idea that to achieve the best medical care they must, at times, be their brothers' keepers, we can expect improvements in drug therapy. This will require that all hospitals develop and activate the machinery for surveillance and that all become accredited by the national accrediting commission. A further step would be to require that every doctor be on the staff of at least one hospital and thus subject to its regulations and susceptible to its educational program.

If insuring good therapy within hospitals is difficult, raising standards of therapy to a reasonable level outside the hospital is a more formidable task. The individual doctor has traditionally been master of his own actions in his office and in the patient's home. And most of the time there is no way to tell what drugs he is prescribing there or why.

But change is in the air here also. The more frequent referral of patients to specialists for consultation or treatment, the rising number of doctors practicing in groups, and the increased use of the hospital to diagnose difficult cases—all of these mean that doctors' actions are open to inspection more frequently than in the past.

Physicians have taken on the obligation of monitoring medical insurance plans. In California physicans who prescribe excessive numbers of drugs, particularly of high-priced drugs, under Blue Shield insurance, Medicare, or Medicaid, come under the scrutiny of a committee of their peers. Where improper practices have been discovered, doctors have been disciplined by their local medical societies.[23]

The organization that can best censure and punish doctors who will not or cannot practice medicine above a minimal standard is the county medical society, the smallest unit of the large network that includes the state medical societies and the AMA. Membership in the county medical society brings many advantages; most doctors prefer to conform to its rules rather than be on the outside. Unfortunately, these societies have tended to look the other way when their members practiced medicine of poor quality, but a concerned public and interested third-party payers are demanding more effective control. It is hoped that the medical societies will respond to the challenge. Here, as in hospitals, the medical profession has been asked to clean the inside of the cup, lest someone else do it for them.

The idea of compulsion in any form is anathema to most doctors. Of all the professions they are probably the most individualistic and independent, and most doctors want to stay that way. At the same time, the practice of medicine is becoming more interdependent as doctors from different specialties work in teams to solve difficult problems and carry out intricate operations. Co-operation is increasingly required as the machinery of medical care is becoming more complex. These trends have required more regulation, most of which has been imposed by the medical profession upon itself, by committees and staff within hospitals, and by national accrediting agencies.

Another kind of regulation was initiated by the American Academy of General Practice, when it set fifty hours of formal postgraduate work during each three-year period as a condition of membership.[24] The College of General Practice of Canada[25] and the Oregon State Medical Society[26] have adopted similar rules. Could not these pioneer efforts be imitated by other national specialty groups so that once a physician had passed his examinations and been certified by a specialty board or the board for family practice, he would be expected in a given number of years to pass examinations in a certain number of courses selected from a specified group? Continued certification by specialty or family practice boards, society memberships, access to hospitals, and even the right to practice might eventually depend upon a doctor's meeting these standards. Utopian? Perhaps. But the rapidity with which medical knowledge is increasing, and the demands of an informed public for the best possible medical care, will require that something of the sort be done. Today's undergraduate medical education would have seemed just as utopian in 1900. Around that time Sir William Osler wrote that the medical school could do no more than teach the student basic principles and methods of work. "These," he continued, "simply start him in the right direction; they do not make him a good practitioner—that is his own affair."[27] Today many would contend that it is society's affair also, and that society must find ways, by encouragement, support, or compulsion, to see that the doctor continues in the right direction.

Up to now such regulation has been left almost entirely to the medical profession. The challenge to raise the standards of their profession remains in the doctors' hands yet a little longer. But as more and more of the medical care is paid for by third parties, private and governmental, they will demand adequate policing by doctors or they will take over the function themselves. *Verbum sapienti!*

I have discussed the impact upon the physician of several factors: advertising generated by million-dollar corporations; regulation by a government agency; the help that he can receive from medical societies, medical journals, and postgraduate courses; and periodic examinations by state licensing boards. But after all of these have had their impact, the doctor is left at the bedside of the patient, and there he faces the moment of truth in which he must make a vital decision. At such times he can either be swayed by suggestion or be ruled by reason. He can weakly yield to the patient's demands for treatment; he can take the opposite pole by asserting his authority; or he can choose a middle course by explaining what he expects to do and thus gain the patient's co-operation.

The doctor needs to make sure that the patient understands the nature of the projected therapy for another reason: patients often do not follow doctors' orders. One study showed that one third[28] and another that four fifths[29] of patients failed to complete a ten-day course of penicillin as prescribed. Among 125 psychiatric patients, 48 per cent failed to take the prescribed drugs, as shown by chemical tests of their urine.[30] Physicians are generally unaware of this. For instance, 22 of 27 physicians overestimated their patients' adherence to a prescribed regimen of antacids.[31]

What is the explanation? Is it mainly that the patient echoes Walt Whitman's sentiments: "I love doctors and hate their medicines"? Perhaps the neglectful one has an unconscious fear of drugs, or perhaps he is merely forgetful. Whatever the reason, the doctor's best remedy is to explain thoroughly to every patient what he expects the medicine to accomplish and why it must be taken in a certain way to bring this about. Explanation alerts the patient to adverse reactions and stimulates him to report them promptly. It gives the patient's hope sustenance on which to feed, so that he does not abandon treatment without reason. And it provides the doctor with a substitute for the prescribing of unneeded drugs. When the patient demands a "shot of penicillin," an explanation of why it is not needed and should not be given is usually gratefully received. What is more, the lesson is lasting, and the extra few minutes spent in the first conversation are saved many times over in the future.

One final point: the strong emphasis on drugs in this chapter does not mean that illness is cured or ameliorated by drugs alone. In some cases they are not required at all. In all cases the sympathetic understanding of the physician is needed. But the doctor does not always know when the patient feels that such understanding is lacking. When he is giving an explanation, he may often uncover hidden doubts and fears that he then has a chance to allay. And he has the opportunity to show that he cares. As one of our greatest medical teachers phrased it:

"Time, sympathy and understanding must be lavishly dispensed, but the reward is to be found in that personal bond which forms the greatest satisfaction of the practice of medicine. One of the essential qualities of the clinician is interest in humanity, for the secret of the care of the patient is in caring for the patient."[32]

*If the trumpet give an uncertain sound, who
shall prepare himself to the battle?*
—CORINTHIANS 14:8

14

The Road Ahead

In the previous chapters we have seen that the process of achieving the best possible health for the American people through drug therapy is deficient at many points. To whom should we look for help? The only realistic answer is: to all who are involved—the drug industry, the medical and allied health professions, the universities, government agencies, and the American public itself. To expect drug-makers to turn philanthropists would be to ignore the laws of economics. To expect doctors alone to solve the problems would be naive. To turn the entire problem over to the federal government for solution would be to sell our birthright.

In a pluralistic society, composed of many groups whose objectives often differ widely, we cannot expect to find a single solution to a complex problem. In this concluding chapter I shall summarize my recommendations for each of the groups involved.

First, let us consider the pharmaceutical industry. We have seen that it is becoming larger and is tending to be absorbed into, and to take on the characteristics of, big business in general. There is a strong possibility that it will lose what is left of its distinctive ethics. Attempts should be made to counteract this by greater professionalization of the personnel in the drug industry. The basic scientists are well integrated into their respective scientific societies, but neither the societies nor the scientists within them have spoken out against the abuses in the industry. As the prestige of scientists continues to increase, they gain the power, and with it the duty, to influence social and economic issues, as physicists have done so effectively with respect to atomic energy.

The physicians in the drug industry could exert influence on the industry if they had a strong organization outside the Pharmaceutical Manufacturers Association, rather than merely a section within it as at present. Detail men also could mobilize their strength and voice their discontents by having an organization of their own. Each of these groups could set up codes of ethics. On the basis of such codes the doctors in industry might force drug companies to give to medical directors a veto power on the marketing of a new drug, and detail men might be able to refuse to convey orally to doctors information that is patently at odds with labeling and printed advertising approved by the FDA.

Professional groups within and without the drug industry should do all they can to convince the executives that industry's best interests would be served by more emphasis on discovering truly new drugs, the marketing of fewer "me-too" drugs, and the communication of consistently accurate information to the practicing physician.

But we can expect only so much from the pharmaceutical companies. One bad actor among a dozen companies may mean that all of them may be forced to adopt his practices or be left behind. Here is where regulation comes in. If it is well conceived and fairly administered, it benefits the more ethical firms, forcing the others to discard their shady practices or have sanctions imposed upon them that will hurt them economically.

Who should do the regulating? In a democracy regulation cannot be accomplished by means of government alone; much of it depends upon the will of the individuals and groups who are regulated and upon the influence of those private organizations that undertake regulation voluntarily. Private regulation depends more upon moral suasion, government regulation upon compulsion; yet each may use both, in different degrees.

Regulation by government has certain obvious strengths. It has the force of law. It can compel obedience. It can subpoena witnesses and thus uncover facts that others cannot find. And government has resources to make regulation as broad and as complete as is required.

In turn, private regulation has its advantages. Although the resources of private groups are limited, sometimes pitifully so, these groups can obtain the volunteer services of professionals. A private group can afford to pioneer. It has less to lose if an experiment fails, and when one succeeds, it can allow government to take over the project and move on to something else. Its flexibility also enables it to take up a new program quickly when an emergency develops. Either governmental or private regulators may be swayed or corrupted so as to favor an individual or group unfairly. In the private agency, those who are concerned can usually prevent this because they are near or in the seat of power. Combating favoritism by a government agency may sometimes depend upon exposing mistakes or improper practices after the fact.

Private agencies may overcome some of their deficiencies by combining with others for a common end. For instance, the American College of Surgeons began to accredit hospitals in 1918. They were so successful that the program grew too big for them, and in 1952 the Joint Commission on Accreditation was formed by the Colleges of Surgeons and Physicians, the AMA, and the American Hospital Association. And as previously mentioned, the naming of drugs was made more effective by the alliance of the AMA, the *USP* (*United States Pharmacopeia*), and the *NF* (*National Formulary*) to form the United States Adopted Names Council.

To make the picture more confusing, regulation does not always stay in the same hands. The most obvious trend is from private to public regulation. An example is the regulation of communicable diseases. The physicians of American cities in colonial times, acting through committees appointed by their medical associations, tried to install certain preventive measures during severe epidemics. In general they were unsuccessful, and eventually city, and later state and federal, governments took over this important function. As has been related, although the AMA was partially effective in curbing excesses in the advertising of drugs to doctors, a more complete job is being done by the federal government since the Drug Amendments Act of 1962.

But the trend in regulation need not go this way. Collaboration between private agencies and government is often a more efficient and rewarding method. This may be formal collaboration; drug standards set up by the *USP* and the *NF* have been recognized in several laws relating to drugs. Another example is the agreement between the commissioner of Food and Drugs and the United States Adopted Names Council.

Or collaboration may be informal. The Joint Council on the Accreditation of Hospitals classifies hospitals; the federal government recognizes the classification when it is allocating funds for construction or the payment of hospital expenses of patients. Likewise, various governmental agencies accept the classifications of specialists made by the various specialty boards. Also, the AMA has co-operated with the FDA, the Federal Trade Commission, and the Post Office Department to try to stamp out quackery.

One would hope that at times functions might be turned back from the government to private hands. This occurs infrequently, but we can see it happening with respect to the state examinations for the practice of medicine. This prerogative was taken over completely by the individual states, creating hardship for doctors moving from one state to another. But gradually over the years a private group, the National Board of Medical Examiners, has developed a program of examinations, which are today accepted by most states in lieu of their own; moreover, in recent years the private group has acquired so much expertise in perfecting examinations that state examining boards are contracting with them to supply questions for the state examinations.

Thus, in spite of the dire warnings of some who believe the federal government is becoming too powerful in the health sphere, much room is left for regulation by private groups. One important condition must be met, however: the private group must have shown that it can do the job. I have outlined in Chapters 8 and 9 certain challenging opportunities for the AMA, the *USP* and the *NF* to move forward into needed areas of regulation. I would couple with this a warning: to expect the government to withhold its hand for any length of time to allow a private agency to build up a regulatory program is to indulge in fantasy. If some private agency does not advance into a needed area of regulation, the government sooner or later will do it. There is room for both private and government regulation. How much will be taken over by government depends on how imaginative, how public-spirited, how broad-visioned, and how aggressive the private agencies are.

So much for private agencies. What can we expect of the FDA? The ingredient most needed to improve its total program is a higher professional stature. In Chapter 11 I suggest several ways in which this can be done. I believe that they should be vigorously pursued.

The Division of Biologics Standards has a smaller and more specialized job to do and seems to be doing it well. I see no reason to change the pattern of its operations. I would hope that the good relations that exist with the FDA could be cemented by a system of continuing committees that would meet at intervals to consider mutual problems and future goals.

With respect to the Congress, I believe that it should probe further into the effects of our present patent systems, the proper allocation of a patent when the research leading to it was supported partly by the government, and the need for changes in the patent laws pertaining to drugs. Because the patent system is becoming increasingly more important both to the general economy and to the public welfare, it should be continuously scrutinized and studied, especially in an area as vital as drugs, and presumably some recommendations for change will result from the scrutiny.

The practicing physician can be helped and stimulated to improve the quality of his therapy by better education in drug therapy during and after medical school and by increasing the advice from and surveillance by peer groups. Also some method should be devised for recertifying the doctor's proficiency at intervals during a lifetime of practice. Implementation of these recommendations devolves upon medical schools, hospitals, and medical societies.

Finally, the general public must be more knowledgeable and more active in the area of drugs. More attention on the part of consumers is needed in every area, but particularly with respect to the protection of the foods they eat, the drugs they take, and the air they breathe, people must be aware of the facts and must be stimulated to action where necessary. The initiative should come from public-spirited citizens, both within and without the health professions, from educators, civic leaders, and informed people generally. Also the FDA should expand its facilities for informing the public of what the problems are and what it is doing about them.

As George S. Shakespeare, Jr., has said:

"I know of no safe depository of the ultimate powers of society but the people themselves; and if we think them not enlightened enough to exercise their control with a wholesome discretion, the remedy is not to take it from them, but to inform their discretion by education."[1]

If these recommendations are followed, there is enough work to keep all the interested groups busy. Hand in hand, all who are concerned with the public good can advance the cause together. The stakes are high: nothing less than the health of the American people.

Notes

INTRODUCTION

1. U.S. Department of Commerce, Bureau of the Census: *Current Industrial Reports. Pharmaceutical Preparations, Except Biologicals, 1965* (Washington, D.C.; 1967), p. 2.
2. Seymour E. Harris: *The Economics of American Medicine* (New York: The Macmillan Company; 1964), p. 73.
3. Estes Kefauver: *In a Few Hands: Monopoly Power in America* (New York: Pantheon Books; 1965).
4. Richard Harris: *The Real Voice* (New York: The Macmillan Company; 1964).
5. Morton Mintz: *By Prescription Only*, rev. ed. (Boston: Beacon Press; 1967). Originally published as *The Therapeutic Nightmare*.
6. Jacques Barzun: *The House of Intellect* (New York: Harper and Brothers; 1959), p. 122.
7. Alan Gregg: *The Furtherance of Medical Research* (New Haven: Yale University Press; 1941), p. 11.

CHAPTER 1

1. Oliver Wendell Holmes: *Medical Essays* (Boston: Houghton Mifflin & Co.; 1891), p. 203.
2. Richard H. Shryock: *The Development of Modern Medicine* (New York: Alfred A. Knopf; 1947), pp. 248–303.
3. G. R. Coatney: "Pitfalls in Discovery: The Chronicle of Chloroquine," *American Journal of Tropical Medicine*, Vol. XII (March 1963), pp. 121–8.
4. *Pharmacopoeia Londinensis of 1618: Reproduced in Facsimile*, with a historical introduction by George Urdang (Madison, Wisconsin: State Historical Society of Wisconsin; 1944).
5. A. Burger: "Approaches to Drug Discovery," *New England Journal of Medicine*, Vol. CCLXX (May 21, 1964), pp. 1098–1101.

6. Paul de Haen: "1960 Pharmaceutical Products Parade," *Drug and Cosmetic Industry*, Vol. LXXXVIII (February 1961), pp. 166–7, 243–8.

7. K. H. Beyer and others: "The Enhancement of the Physiological Economy of Penicillin in Dogs by the Simultaneous Administration of Para-Aminohippuric Acid II," *Journal of Pharmacology and Experimental Therapeutics*, Vol. LXXXII (December 1944), pp. 310–23.

8. H. F. Dowling and T. J. Abernethy: "The Treatment of Pneumococcus Pneumonia: A Comparison of the Results Obtained with Specific Serum and with Sulfapyridine," *American Journal of the Medical Sciences*, Vol. CXCIX (January 1940), pp. 55–62; H. F. Dowling and M. H. Lepper: "The Effect of Antibiotics (Penicillin, Aureomycin, and Terramycin) on the Fatality Rate and Incidence of Complications in Pneumococcic Pneumonia. A Comparison with Other Methods of Therapy," *American Journal of the Medical Sciences*, Vol. CCXXII (October 1951), pp. 396–403.

CHAPTER 2

1. W. D. M. Paton: "The Early Days of Pharmacology, with Special Reference to the Nineteenth Century," in F. N. L. Poynter, ed.: *Chemistry in the Service of Medicine* (London: Pitman Medical Publishing Co., Ltd.; 1963), p. 86.

2. Suellen Muldoon, ed.: *A.A.M.C. Directory* (Evanston, Illinois: Association of American Medical Colleges; 1968).

3. U.S. Department of Health, Education and Welfare, Public Health Service: *Resources for Medical Research. Report No. 8: Trends in R & D Manpower in the Pharmaceutical Industry 1959–65 and 1968* (Washington, D.C.: Government Printing Office; 1966), pp. 2, 11.

4. J. B. Blake: "Scientific Institutions Since the Renaissance: Their Role in Medical Research," *Proceedings of the American Philosophical Society*, Vol. CI (February 1957), pp. 31–62.

5. W. W. Oliver: *The Man Who Lived for Tomorrow: A Biography of William Hallock Park, M.D.* (New York: E. P. Dutton; 1941).

6. Ralph Chester Williams: *The United States Public Health Service 1798–1950* (Washington, D.C.: Commissioned Officers Association of the Public Health Service; 1951), pp. 184, 196–8, 205, 223.

7. U.S. Department of Health, Education and Welfare: *Advancement of Knowledge for the Nation's Health. A Report to the President on the Research Programs of the National Institutes of Health* (Washington, D.C.: Government Printing Office, 1967), p. 55.

8. Letter to the author from Kenneth M. Endicott, National Cancer Institute, April 9, 1969.

9. U.S. Department of Health, Education and Welfare: *Advancement of Knowledge*, op. cit., pp. 90–108, 110–16, 169–70.

10. G. R. Coatney: "Pitfalls in a Discovery: The Chronicle of Chloroquine," *American Journal of Tropical Medicine*, Vol. XII (March 1963), pp. 121–8.

11. *Hospital Tribune*, November 20, 1967, p. 18.

12. L. I. Dublin, A. J. Lotka, and M. Spiegelman: *Length of Life*, rev. ed. (New York: The Ronald Press Co.; 1949), p. 42.

13. Ralph Waldo Emerson: "Society and Solitude," in *Concord Papers and Other Essays* (New York: E. P. Dutton; [n.d.]), p. 105.

14. Glenn Sonnedecker: "The Rise of Drug Manufacture in America," *Emory University Quarterly*, Vol. XXI (Summer 1965), pp. 73–87.

15. Ibid., p. 77.

16. "Now 25 Oldest Drug Houses," *Drug and Cosmetic Industry*, Vol. LXX (January 1952), p. 29.

17. Oliver, op. cit., p. 210.

18. H. Kogan: *The Long White Line: The Story of the Abbott Laboratories*, (New York: Random House; 1963), pp. 90–4.

19. Richard H. Shryock: *American Medical Research, Past and Present* (New York: Commonwealth Fund; 1947), pp. 58, 161–2.

20. Tom Mahoney: *The Merchants of Life. An Account of the American Pharmaceutical Industry* (New York: Harper and Brothers; 1959), pp. 213–4.

21. H. F. Dowling: "Broad-Spectrum Antibiotics After Ten Years," *Medical Annals of the District of Columbia*, Vol. XXVIII (December 1959), pp. 695–7.

22. "Who Killed Cock Robin?" editorial, *American Journal of Public Health*, Vol. XXXIV (June 1944), pp. 658–9.

23. A. N. Richards: "Production of Penicillin in the United States (1941–1946)," *Nature*, Vol. CCI (February 1964), pp. 441–5.

24. U.S. Department of Health, Education and Welfare: *Advancement of Knowledge*, op. cit., pp. 11–19.

25. Ibid., pp. 53–4.

26. U.S. Department of Health, Education, and Welfare: *Task Force on Prescription Drugs. The Drug Makers and the Drug Distributors* (Washington, D.C.: Government Printing Office, December 1968), p. 16.

27. *Drug Trade News*, December 30, 1968, p. 15.

28. U.S. House of Representatives, Committee on Government Operations, Subcommittee, 88th Cong., 2nd Sess.: *Hearings on Drug Safety* (1964), Pt. 1, p. 313.

29. Ibid., p. 302.

CHAPTER 3

1. Harvey Brooks: "Applied Science and Technological Progress," *Science*, Vol. CLVI (June 30, 1967), pp. 1706–12.

2. A. M. Richards: "Production of Penicillin in the United States (1941–1946)," *Nature*, Vol. CCI (February 1, 1964), pp. 441–5.

3. United States Tariff Commission: *Synthetic Organic Chemicals, United States Production and Sales, 1964, T. C. Publication 167* (Washington, D.C.: Government Printing Office; 1965).

4. J. T. Connor: "The Functions of the Pharmaceutical Industry in Our Society," in Paul Talalay, ed.: *Drugs in Our Society* (Baltimore: Johns Hopkins Press; 1964), p. 119.

5. Carl A. Dragstedt: "Oral Medication with Preparations for Prolonged Action," *The Journal of the American Medical Association*, Vol. CLXVIII (November 22, 1958), pp. 1652–8.

6. Ralph G. Smith: "How Safe Are Drugs? The Viewpoint of the Food and Drug Administration," *Journal of New Drugs*, Vol. VI (January–February 1966), pp. 62–8.

7. R. S. Cowles: "Quality Control in the Manufacture of Drugs," *Bio-medical Purview*, Vol. III (Summer 1963), pp. 51–8.

8. E. L. Meyers: *FDC Reports, Drugs and Cosmetics. "Textbook"*

on *Quality Control in Drug Production* from FDA, industry papers during University of Wisconsin seminar (Washington: FDC Reports, Inc.; 1965), p. 27.

9. U.S. House of Representatives, Committee on Government Operations, Subcommittee, 88th Cong., 2nd Sess.: *Hearings on Drug Safety* (1964), Pt. 1, p. 282.

10. "Financial Data on 290 Drug Field Companies Shown," *Drug Trade News*, September 26, 1966, p. 14.

11. *Facts about Pharmacy and Pharmaceuticals* (New York: Health News Institute, Inc.; 1958), p. 39.

12. W. W. Oliver: *The Man Who Lived for Tomorrow: A Biography of William Hallock Park, M.D.* (New York: E. P. Dutton and Company; 1941), p. 63.

13. G. Zbinden: "The Significance of Pharmacologic Screening Tests in the Preclinical Safety Evaluation of New Drugs," *Journal of New Drugs*, Vol. VI (January–February 1966), pp. 1–8.

14. T. Koppanyi and M. A. Avery: "Species Differences and the Clinical Trial of New Drugs: A Review," *Clinical Pharmacology and Therapeutics*, Vol. VII (March–April 1966), p. 250.

15. J. T. Litchfield, Jr.: "Evaluation of the Safety of New Drugs by Means of Tests in Animals," Symposium on Clinical Drug Evaluation and Human Pharmacology: Part XVI, *Clinical Pharmacology and Therapeutics*, Vol. III (September–October 1962), p. 665.

16. Zbinden: loc. cit.

17. B. B. Brodie: "Difficulties in Extrapolating Data on Metabolism of Drugs from Animal to Man," *Clinical Pharmacology and Therapeutics*, Vol. III (May–June 1962), pp. 374–80.

18. *Report of the Commission on Drug Safety* (Washington, D.C.: Commission on Drug Safety; 1964), pp. 27–65.

19. Ibid., pp. 45–6, 56–8. Also, *Report of the Conference of Prenatal Effects of Drugs* (Chicago: Commission on Drug Safety; 1963).

CHAPTER 4

1. Wyndham B. Blanton: *Medicine in Virginia in the Eighteenth Century* (Richmond, Virginia: Garrett and Massie, Inc.; 1931), pp. 305–6.

2. *Drug Research Reports*, Vol. XI (February 8, 1968), pp. 16–18.

3. E. R. Beckerstaff and J. McD. Holmes: "Cerebral Arterial Insufficiency and Oral Contraceptives," *British Medical Journal*, Vol. I (March 25, 1967), pp. 726–9.
4. S. H. Ferebee, F. W. Mount, and G. W. Comstock: "The Use of Chemotherapy as a Prophylactic Measure in Tuberculosis," *Annals of the New York Academy of Sciences*, Vol. CVI (February 28, 1963), pp. 151–6.
5. John Rowan Wilson: *Margin of Safety* (Garden City, New York: Doubleday and Company, Inc.: 1963), p. 86.
6. Harry F. Dowling: "Human Dissection and Experimentation with Drugs," *The Journal of the American Medical Association*, Vol. CCII (December 25, 1967), pp. 1132–5; "The Dilemma of Human Experimentation with Drugs: A Historical Perspective," *Journal of Clinical Pharmacology*, Vol. VII (September–October 1967), pp. 248–50.
7. Harry F. Dowling: "Human Experimentation in Infectious Diseases," *The Journal of the American Medical Association*, Vol. CXCVIII (November 28, 1964), pp. 997–9.
8. Drug Research Reports, Vol. 12, No. 32 (Supplement), August 6, 1969, pp. S–34—S–45.
9. "The Relation of the Clinical Investigator to the Patient, Pharmaceutical Industry and Federal Agencies," Fourth Bethesda Conference of the American College of Cardiology, August 27 and 28, 1966, *American Journal of Cardiology*, Vol. XIX (June 1967), p. 901.
10. William B. Bean: "A Testament of Duty," *Journal of Laboratory and Clinical Medicine*, Vol. XXXIX (January 1952), pp. 3–9.
11. Richard P. Bergen: "Healthy Subjects in Clinical Investigation," *The Journal of the American Medical Association*, Vol. CCIII (February 26, 1968), pp. 369–70.
12. Letter from William H. Stewart, Surgeon General, United States Public Health Service, to heads of institutions conducting research with Public Health Service grants, February 8, 1966.
13. I. Ladimer: "Symposium on the Study of Drugs in Man. I. Medical Experimentation: Legal Consideration," *Clinical Pharmacology and Therapeutics*, Vol. I, (September–October 1959), pp. 674–82.
14. Harry F. Dowling: "Responsibility for Testing Drugs in Humans," *The Journal of the American Medical Association*, Vol. CLXXX-

VII (January 18, 1964), pp. 212–15. Another viewpoint is expressed in Louis Lasagna: "Clinical Pharmacology: Present Status and Future Development," *Science*, Vol. CLII (April 15, 1966), pp. 388–91.

15. Ferebee, Mount, and Comstock: loc cit., pp. 151–6.
16. D. Wheatley: "The General Practitioner Research Group," *Clinical Pharmacology and Therapeutics*, Vol. IV (July–August 1963), pp. 542–7.
17. U.S. Senate, Committee on Government Operations, Subcommittee on Reorganization and International Organizations, 89th Cong., 2nd Sess.: *Interagency Drug Coordination* (1966), pp. 224–5.
18. A. B. Hill: "The Experimental Approach in Preventive Medicine: Controlled Trials of Vaccines," *Journal of the Royal Institute of Public Health and Hygiene*, Vol. XXI (July 1958), pp. 185–208.
19. Henry K. Beecher: "Qualitative Effects of Drugs on the Mind," in Paul Talalay, ed.: *Drugs in Our Society* (Baltimore: The Johns Hopkins Press; 1964), pp. 82–3.
20. O. B. Ross, Jr.: "Use of Controls in Medical Research," *The Journal of the American Medical Association*, Vol. CXLV (January 13, 1951), pp. 72–5.
21. "Nitrate Therapy for Angina Pectoris Still Debated After 100 Years," *The Journal of the American Medical Association*, Vol. CXCIX (March 6, 1967), pp. 35–6.
22. René Dubos: *Miracle of Health: Utopias, Progress, and Biological Change* (New York: Harper and Brothers; 1959).
23. John Lewis: "Drug Evaluation by Council on Drugs," *The Journal of the American Medical Association*, Vol. CLXXXV (July 27, 1963), pp. 256–8.
24. U.S. Senate, Committee on Government Operations, Subcommittee on Reorganization and International Organizations, 88th Cong., 1st Sess.: *Hearings on Interagency Coordination in Drug Research and Regulation* (1963), Pt. 3, pp. 781–2.
25. U.S. Senate, Committee on Government Operations, Subcommittee on Reorganization and International Organizations, 88th Cong., 1st Sess.: *Hearings on Interagency Coordination in Drug Research and Regulation, Hearings* (1964), Pt. 6, pp. 3197–202.
26. Ibid., Pt. 4, p. 1682.
27. Richard H. Shryock: *The Development of Modern Medicine: An*

Interpretation of the Social and Scientific Factors Involved (New York: Alfred A. Knopf; 1947), pp. 159–60.

28. Ibid., pp. 138–40.

29. S. Schor and I. Karten: "Statistical Evaluation of Manuscripts," *The Journal of the American Medical Association*, Vol. CXCV (March 28, 1966), pp. 1123–8.

30. W. Modell and R. W. House: "Factors Influencing Clinical Evaluation of Drugs with Special Reference to the Double-Blind Technique: Report to the Council on Drugs," *The Journal of the American Medical Association*, Vol. CLXVII (August 30, 1958), pp. 2190–8. This article gives many excellent suggestions regarding the problems and pitfalls accompanying the study of drugs in humans.

CHAPTER 5

1. U.S. Senate, Committee on the Judiciary, Subcommittee on Antitrust and Monopoly, 87th Cong., 1st Sess.: *Hearings on the Drug Industry Antitrust Act* (1961), Pt. 1, p. 15.

2. Richard Harris: *The Real Voice* (New York: The Macmillan Company; 1964), p. 90.

3. E. P. Learned and others: *Business Policy: Text and Cases* (Homewood, Illinois: Richard D. Irwin, Inc.; 1965), p. 541.

4. "Broad Screening for Pinpoint Therapy," *Medical World News*, Vol. VII (November 11, 1966), pp. 43–6, 130–8.

5. U.S. Department of Commerce, Bureau of the Census: "Pharmaceutical Preparations, Except Biologicals, 1967," *Current Industrial Reports* (Washington, D.C.: Government Printing Office; December 4, 1968), p. 2.

6. *Drug Trade News*, January 31, 1966, p. 16.

7. U.S. Department of Commerce, Bureau of the Census: "1963 Industry Statistics: Drugs," *Census of Manufacturers* (Washington, D.C.: Government Printing Office; 1966) p. 7.

8. E. C. Robins: *Making Today's Medicines with Integrity . . . Seeking Tomorrow's with Persistence: The Story of A. H. Robins Company* (Princeton: Princeton University Press; 1966), pp. 12–13.

9. U.S. Senate, Committee on the Judiciary, Subcommittee on Anti-trust and Monopoly, 87th Cong., 1st Sess.: *Study of Administered Prices in the Drug Industry* (1961), p. 77.

10. R. J. DeSalvo and M. Musulin: "Drug and Cosmetic Mergers," *Drug and Cosmetic Industry*, Vol. XCVIII (June 1966), pp. 53–5, 171–4.

11. "The Fortune Directory of the 500 Largest U.S. Industrial Corporations," *Fortune Magazine*, June 15, 1968, pp. 186–220.

12. *Drug Trade News*, February 10, 1969, p. 1.

13. Pharmaceutical Manufacturers Association: "Administrative Officers of the Member Firms of the Pharmaceutical Manufacturers Association" (Washington: July 1966).

14. U.S. Senate, Select Committee on Small Business, Subcommittee on Monopoly, 90th Cong., 1st and 2nd Sess.: *Hearings on Competitive Problems in the Drug Industry* (1968), Pt. 5, p. 2061.

15. U.S. Department of Justice: *Merger Guidelines* (Washington, D.C.: May 30, 1968), p. 2.

16. "Maneuvering the Body's Chemicals for Therapy," *Medical World News*, December 16, 1966, pp. 39–43, 122–7, 130–1, 135.

17. Sheldon Zalaznick: "Bitter Pills for the Drugmakers," *Fortune*, July 1968, pp. 83–5, 148–51.

18. U.S. Senate, Committee on the Judiciary, Subcommittee on Anti-trust and Monopoly, 87th Cong., 1st Sess.: *Hearings on the Drug Industry Antitrust Act* (1962), Pt. 4, pp. 2516–34.

19. Jesse W. Markham: "Economic Incentives and Progress in the Drug Industry," in Paul Talalay, ed.: *Drugs in Our Society* (Baltimore: Johns Hopkins Press; 1964), p. 169.

20. U.S. Senate, Committee on the Judiciary, Subcommittee on Anti-trust and Monopoly, 87th Cong., 1st Sess.: *Study of Administered Prices in the Drug Industry* (1961), pp. 66–8.

21. Ibid., pp. 69–71.

22. Ministry of Health: *Final Report of the Committee on Cost of Prescribing* (London: Her Majesty's Stationery Office, 1959), p. 68.

23. P. R. Garai: "Advertising and Promotion of Drugs," in Tallay: op. cit., p. 194.

24. John Kenneth Galbraith: *American Capitalism: The Concept of Countervailing Power*, rev. ed. (Cambridge, Massachusetts: Riverside Press; 1956), p. 43.

CHAPTER 6

1. U.S. Senate, Select Committee on Small Business, Subcommittee on Monopoly, 90th Cong., 1st Sess.: *Hearings on Competitive Problems in the Drug Industry* (1967), Pt. 1, p. 202; 1st and 2nd Sess. (1968), Pt. 5, p. 1710.
2. Morton Mintz: "Drug Pricing Case Has Wide Impact," *Washington Post*, January 21, 1968, p. E10.
3. Seymour E. Harris: *The Economics of American Medicine* (New York: The Macmillan Company; 1964), p. 103.
4. U.S. Senate: *Hearings on Competitive Problems* (1967), op. cit., p. 204.
5. U. S. Senate: *Hearings on Competitive Problems* (1968), op. cit., p. 1713.
6. Ibid., p. 1937.
7. Ibid., pp. 1667–90.
8. Ibid., p. 2056.
9. Ibid., pp. 1819, 1820, 1815.
10. Ibid., pp. 1897, 1900, 1881.
11. U.S. Senate, Committee on the Judiciary, Subcommittee on Antitrust and Monopoly, 87th Cong., 1st Sess.: *Hearings on Drug Industry Antitrust Act* (1962), Pt. 4, p. 2054.
12. Richard Burack: *The Handbook of Prescription Drugs. Official Names, Prices and Sources for Patient and Doctor* (New York: Pantheon Books; 1967), pp. 124–5.
13. Pharmaceutical Manufacturers Association: "The Importance of Manufacturer Identification" (Washington, D.C.: October 1965), p. 9.
14. Burack: op. cit., p. 84.
15. Ibid., pp. 36–71.
16. Ibid., p. 135.
17. Ibid., p. 155.
18. U.S. Department of Health, Education, and Welfare, Office of the Secretary: *Task Force on Prescription Drugs, Second Interim Report and Recommendations* (Washington, D.C.: August 30, 1968), p. 76.
19. U.S. Senate: *Hearings on Competitive Problems* (1967), op. cit., pp. 409–10.

20. U.S. Department of Health, Education, and Welfare, Office of the Secretary: *Task Force on Prescription Drugs: Final Report* (Washington, D.C.: February 7, 1969), p. 33.

21. U.S. Senate, Committee on the Judiciary, Subcommittee on Antitrust and Monopoly, 87th Cong., 1st Sess.: *Study of Administered Prices in the Drug Industry* (1961), pp. 106–7.

22. U.S. Senate: *Hearings on Competitive Problems* (1968), op. cit., p. 2066.

23. U.S. Department of Health, Education and Welfare: *Task Force: Final Report*, op. cit., p. 15.

24. P. R. Garai: "Advertising and Promotion of Drugs," in Paul Talalay, ed.: *Drugs in Our Society* (Baltimore: The Johns Hopkins Press; 1964), p. 199.

25. Burack: op. cit., pp. 74–158.

26. C. A. Blick: "The Defense Supply Agency Takes a Fresh Look at Drug Procurement," Address delivered at the Nineteenth Annual Luncheon, National Pharmaceutical Council (New York City: December 11, 1963).

27. U.S. Senate: *Hearings on Drug Industry Antitrust Act*, op. cit., p. 2235.

CHAPTER 7

1. P. R. Garai: "Advertising and Promotion of Drugs," in Paul Talalay, ed.: *Drugs in Our Society* (Baltimore: The Johns Hopkins Press; 1964), pp. 192, 199.

2. U.S. Senate, Committee on the Judiciary, Subcommittee on Antitrust and Monopoly, 87th Cong., 1st Sess.: *Study of Administered Prices in the Drug Industry* (1961), p. 157.

3. "Apothecaries Undismayed," editorial, *New England Journal of Medicine*, Vol. CCLXIX (August 29, 1963), pp. 480–1.

4. U.S. Senate: *Study of Administered Prices*, op. cit., p. 157.

5. Garai: in Talalay: op. cit., p. 191.

6. C. D. May: "Selling Drugs by 'Educating' Physicians," *Journal of Medical Education*, Vol. XXXVI (January 1961), pp. 1–23.

7. Ibid., p. 3.

8. U.S. Senate, Committee on Governmental Operations, Subcom-

mittee on Reorganization and International Organizations, 87th Cong., 2nd Sess.: *Hearings on Interagency Coordination in Drug Research and Regulation* (1963), Pt. 3, p. 993.

9. S. Garb: "The Reaction of Medical Students to Drug Advertising," *New England Journal of Medicine*, Vol. CCLIX (July 17, 1958), pp. 121–3.

10. "Industry and Profession," editorial, *Lancet*, Vol. II, (August 19, 1961), pp. 411–12.

11. R. W. D. Turner: "Letters to the Editor," *Lancet*, Vol. II (November 3, 1956), p. 943.

12. Bernard Barber: *Drugs and Society* (New York: Russell Sage Foundation; 1967), p. 55.

13. U.S. Senate, Committee on the Judiciary, Subcommittee on Antitrust and Monopoly, 86th Cong., 2nd Sess.: *Hearings on Administered Prices* (1960), Pt. 19, p. 10368.

14. Sheldon Zalaznick: "Bitter Pills for the Drugmakers," *Fortune*, July 1968, pp. 83–5, 148–51.

15. U.S. Senate, Select Committee on Small Business, Subcommittee on Monopoly, 90th Cong., 1st and 2nd Sess., *Hearings on Competitive Problems in the Drug Industry* (1968), Pt. 6, p. 2583.

16. Garai: in Talalay: op. cit., p. 195.

17. U.S. Senate: *Study of Administered Prices* (1961), op. cit., p. 173.

18. R. A. Bauer and M. G. Field: "Ironic Contrast: U.S. and U.S.S.R. Drug Industries," *Harvard Business Review*, Vol. XL (September–October 1962), pp. 89–97.

19. M. I. Goldman: "Product Differentiation and Advertising: Some Lessons from Soviet Experience," *Journal of Political Economy*, Vol. LXVIII (August 1960), pp. 346–57.

20. "France: Long Strict Drug Controls," *Drug Trade News*, May 5, 1969, p. 36.

CHAPTER 8

1. Chalmers L. Gemmill: "Letter of the First Century A. D. of Pharmacologic Interest," *Bulletin of the History of Medicine*, Vol. XXXIX (January–February 1965), pp. 82–3.

2. William Brown: *Pharmacopoeia Simpliciorum et Efficaciorum* (Philadelphia: Styner and Cist; 1778).

3. E. F. Cook: "The Architects of U.S.P. Destiny," in *Program of the Unveiling and Dedication of a Painting by Robert Thom* (New York: U. S. Pharmacopeia; May 1, 1957), pp. 10, 11.

4. *The Pharmacopeia of the United States of America*, 17th ed. (New York: The United States Pharmacopeial Convention Incorporated; 1965), p. xxiv.

5. J. F. Hoge: "An Appraisal of the New Drug and Cosmetic Legislation from the Viewpoint of Those Industries," *Law and Contemporary Problems*, Vol. VI (Winter 1939), pp. 111–28.

6. G. L. Baker: "Statistics on Occurrence of USP and NF Chemicals in Prescriptions," *Journal of the American Pharmaceutical Association*, Vol. IV (March 1964) pp. 116–17.

7. E. G. Feldmann: "Biopharmaceutics and Drug Standards," *American Journal of Hospital Pharmacy*, Vol. XXV (March 1968), pp. 110–19.

8. U.S. Senate, Select Committee on Small Business, Subcommittee on Monopoly, 90th Cong., 1st Sess.: *Hearings on Competitive Problems in the Drug Industry* (1967), Pt. 1, pp. 401–2.

9. A good history of the early editions of the *NF* is given in *The National Formulary*, 8th rev. (Washington, D.C.: American Pharmaceutical Association; 1946).

10. U.S. Senate: *Hearings on Competitive Problems*, op. cit., p. 416.

CHAPTER 9

1. Morris A. Fishbein: *History of the American Medical Association 1847–1947* (Philadelphia: W. B. Saunders Co.; 1947), p. 30.

2. Ibid., pp. 112, 115, 152, 156.

3. P. Maxwell Foshay: in ibid., p. 198.

4. "Reports to the House of Delegates," *The Journal of the American Medical Association*, Vol. XLV (July 22, 1905), p. 265.

5. "The American Medical Association: Its Friends and Its Enemies," editorial, *The Journal of the American Medical Association*, Vol. XLVII (September 8, 1906), pp. 778–9.

6. "Scientific Work Misrepresented and Commercialized," *The*

Journal of the American Medical Association, Vol. XLV (September 23, 1905), p. 934.

7. Fishbein: op. cit., p. 265.

8. "Wine of Cardui: A Pillar of the Church and His 'Patent-Medicine' Tipple," *The Journal of the American Medical Association*, Vol. LXII (April 11, 1914), p. 1186; and Fishbein: op. cit., p. 285.

9. "A Review of the Food and Drug Situation," editorial, *The Journal of the American Medical Association*, Vol. LXV (July 24, 1915), pp. 334–5.

10. Council on Pharmacy and Chemistry, American Medical Association: *New and Nonofficial Remedies* (Chicago: American Medical Association; 1926), p. 19.

11. "Report of the Board of Trustees," *The Journal of the American Medical Association*, Vol. LXXVI (June 11, 1921), pp. 1657–60.

12. "Report of the Board of Trustees," *Proceedings of the House of Delegates of the American Medical Association* (June 9–13, 1924), p. 12.

13. "Report of the Board of Trustees," *Proceedings of the House of Delegates of the American Medical Association* (June 2–6, 1941), p. 13.

14. A. Smith and W. Van Winkle: "The Cost of Clinical Research," *The Journal of the American Medical Association*, Vol. CXXXIII (January 4, 1947), pp. 30–1.

15. "Report of the Board of Trustees," *Proceedings of the House of Delegates of the American Medical Association* (December 6–9, 1949), p. 14.

16. H. L. Kretschmer: "The Teaching of Drug Therapy," *The Journal of the American Medical Association*, Vol. CXXV (June 3, 1944), pp. 326–7.

17. "Report of the Board of Trustees," *Proceedings of the House of Delegates of the American Medical Association* (December 9–11, 1946), p. 3.

18. "Address of President Dr. E. L. Bortz," *Proceedings of the House of Delegates of the American Medical Association* (January 5–6, 1948), p. 3.

19. E. L. Sevringhaus: "Interdependence of the Medical Profession and the Pharmaceutical Industry," *The Journal of the American Medical Association*, Vol. CLII (August 15, 1953), pp. 1522–5.

20. "Report of the Board of Trustees," *Proceedings of the House of Delegates of the American Medical Association* (November 29–December 2, 1954), p. 43.

21. "Report of the Board of Trustees," *The Journal of the American Medical Association*, Vol. XLV (July 22, 1905), p. 264.

22. "The American Medical Association—Its Policies and Its Work," editorial, *The Journal of the American Medical Association*, Vol. LIV (March 5, 1910), pp. 796–7.

23. "Report of the Board of Trustees," *Proceedings of the House of Delegates of the American Medical Association* (June 3–6, 1912), p. 7.

24. "Report of the Board of Trustees," *Proceedings of the House of Delegates of the American Medical Association* (April 19–23, 1926), p. 6.

25. "Report of the Board of Trustees," *Proceedings of the House of Delegates of the American Medical Association* (May 22–26, 1922), p. 9.

26. "Address of President-Elect Rock Sleyster," *Proceedings of the House of Delegates of the American Medical Association* (May 15–19, 1939), p. 5.

27. Council on Pharmacy and Chemistry, American Medical Association: "A Statement," *The Journal of the American Medical Association*, Vol. CXXXVI (February 7, 1948), p. 399.

28. U.S. Senate, Committee on the Judiciary, Subcommittee on Antitrust and Monopoly, 87th Cong., 1st Sess.: *Hearings on Drug Industry Antitrust Act* (1961), Pt. 1, p. 129.

29. J. W. Richardson, American Medical Association, personal communication, February 26, 1968.

30. Council on Pharmacy and Chemistry, American Medical Association: "New Program of Operation for Evaluation of Drugs," *The Journal of the American Medical Association*, Vol. CLVIII (July 30, 1955), pp. 1170–1.

31. U.S. Senate: *Hearings on Drug Industry Antitrust Act*, op. cit., p. 126; Pt. 2, p. 530.

32. Council on Pharmacy and Chemistry, American Medical Association, Report to the Council: "Blood Dyscrasias Associated with Chlorpromazine Therapy," *The Journal of the American Medical Association*, Vol. CLX (January 28, 1956), p. 287; Council on Drugs, American Medical Association, Report to the Council:

"Blood Dyscrasias Associated with Chloramphenicol (Chloromycetin) Therapy," *The Journal of the American Medical Association*, Vol. CLXXII (April 30, 1960), pp. 2044–5; C. M. Huguley, Jr., A. J. Erslev, and D. E. Bergsagel: "Drug-Related Blood Dyscrasias," *The Journal of the American Medical Association*, Vol. CLXXVII (July 8, 1961), pp. 23–6.

33. W. R. Best: "Drug-Associated Blood Dyscrasias," *The Journal of the American Medical Association*, Vol. CLXXXV (July 27, 1963), pp. 286–90.

34. "USAN, FDA Compromise, Agreement on Drug Names," *The Journal of the American Medical Association*, Vol. CCI (August 21, 1967), p. 1.

35. "Report of the Board of Trustees," *The Journal of the American Medical Association*, Vol. XLV (July 22, 1905), p. 265.

36. "The Pure Food Law," editorial, *The Journal of the American Medical Association*, Vol. XLVII (July 14, 1906), pp. 116–17.

37. "State Pure Food and Drug Legislation Needed," editorial, *The Journal of the American Medical Association*, Vol. XLVII (August 4, 1906), pp. 365–6.

38. "Report of the Board of Trustees," *The Journal of the American Medical Association*, Vol. XLV (July 22, 1905), p. 265.

39. James G. Burrow: *AMA, Voice of American Medicine* (Baltimore: The Johns Hopkins Press; 1963), p. 117.

40. "Ambruster, Rusby—and Ergot," *The Journal of the American Medical Association*, Vol. XCV (September 6, 1930), pp. 722–9; C. O. Jackson: "The Ergot Controversy: Prologue to the 1938 Food, Drug and Cosmetic Act," *Journal of the History of Medicine*, Vol. XXIII (July 1968), p. 248.

41. "The Tugwell-Copeland Pure Food, Drugs and Cosmetic Bill," *The Journal of the American Medical Association*, Vol. CII (March 3, 1934), p. 696.

42. "New Food and Drugs Legislation," *The Journal of the American Medical Association*, Vol. CIV (January 12, 1935), p. 124.

43. "The Emasculated New Food and Drug Bill," *The Journal of the American Medical Association*, Vol. CVI (May 30, 1936), p. 1902.

44. "Federal Food and Drug Bill," editorial, *The Journal of the American Medical Association*, Vol. CX (April 23, 1938), pp. 1370–2.

45. "Report of the Board of Trustees," *Proceedings of the House of Delegates of the American Medical Association* (June 8–12, 1942), p. 12.
46. W. Van Winkle, Jr., and others: "Laboratory and Clinical Appraisal of a New Drug," *The Journal of the American Medical Association*, Vol. CXXVI (December 9, 1944), pp. 958–61.
47. U.S. Senate: *Hearings on Drug Industry Antitrust Act*, op. cit., Pt. 2, p. 999.
48. Ibid., p. 1010.
49. "Report of the Board of Trustees," *Proceedings of the House of Delegates of the American Medical Association* (November 29–Dcember 2, 1954), p. 42.
50. U.S. Senate: *Hearings on Drug Industry Antitrust Act*, op. cit., Pt. 2, p. 1009.
51. "Report of the Board of Trustees," *Proceedings of the House of Delegates of the American Medical Association* (April 26–30, 1920), p. 8.
52. Burrow: op. cit., p. 128.
53. U.S. Senate: *Hearings on Drug Industry Antitrust Act*, op. cit., Pt. 2, p. 491.
54. Ibid., Pt. 1, pp. 125, 129.
55. Ibid., pp. 114, 140.
56. Ibid., pp. 129, 135–6.
57. Ibid., p. 104.
58. Ibid., p. 114.
59. Ibid., pp. 113, 120.
60. Letter from Morris Fishbein to Perrin H. Long, December 11, 1953.
61. U.S. Senate: *Hearings on Drug Industry Antitrust Act*, op. cit., Pt. 1, p. 91.
62. Council on Pharmacy and Chemistry, American Medical Association: "Larodon 'Roche' Not Acceptable for NNR," *The Journal of the American Medical Association*, Vol. CIX (July 17, 1937), p. 209.
63. "Minutes of the House of Delegates," *The Journal of the American Medical Association*, Vol. XLV (July 22, 1905), p. 265.
64. Council on Drugs, American Medical Association: "AMA Drug Evaluations, A New Book on Drugs," *The Journal of the American*

Medical Association, Vol. CCIV (May 20, 1968), pp. 702–10.

65. U.S. Senate: *Hearings on Drug Industry Antitrust Act*, op. cit., Pt. 1, p. 131.

66. "AMA's Expenditures Up, Gross Revenue Down," *AMA News*, May 19, 1969, p. 8.

67. Burrow: op. cit., pp. 354–85.

68. Ibid., p. 146.

69. Richard Harris: "Annals of Legislation, Medicare II. More Than a Lot of Statistics," *The New Yorker*, (July 9, 1966), pp. 30–8, 41–4, 49–51, 55–77.

70. G. E. Farrar: "*Nolle Nocere*: The Responsibility of the Pharmaceutical Industry," *Annals of Internal Medicine*, Vol. L (March 1959), p. 834.

71. Council on Dental Therapeutics, American Dental Association: *Accepted Dental Remedies* (Chicago: American Dental Association; 1934).

72. *ADA Audit* (Chicago: American Dental Association; 1967), p. 20.

CHAPTER 10

1. E. W. Stieb and G. Sonnedecker: *Drug Adulteration. Detection and Control in Nineteenth Century Britain* (Madison, Wisconsin: University of Wisconsin Press; 1966), p. 117–18 et seq.

2. O. E. Anderson, Jr.: *The Health of a Nation. Harvey W. Wiley and the Fight for Pure Food* (Chicago: University of Chicago Press; 1958), pp. 72–4.

3. Ibid., p. 156.

4. C. C. Regier: "The Struggle for Federal Food and Drugs Legislation," *Law and Contemporary Problems*, Vol. I, (December 1933), pp. 3–15.

5. James Harvey Young: "Social History of American Drug Regulation," in Paul Talalay, ed.: *Drugs in Our Society* (Baltimore: The Johns Hopkins Press; 1964), p. 217.

6. Anderson: op. cit., p. 236.

7. Cavers, D. F.: "The Food, Drug and Cosmetic Act of 1938: Its Legislative History and Its Substantive Provisions," *Law and Contemporary Problems*, Vol. VI (Winter 1939), pp. 2–42.

8. James Harvey Young: "The Elixir Sulfanilamide Disaster," *Emory University Quarterly*, Vol. XIV (December 1958), pp. 230–7.
9. Ibid., p. 231.
10. U.S. Senate, Committee on Government Operations, Subcommittee on Reorganization and International Organizations, 87th Cong., 2nd Sess.: *Hearings on Interagency Coordination in Drug Research and Regulations* (1963), Pt. 2, p. 461.
11. W. F. Janssen: "FDA Since 1938: The Major Trends and Developments," *Journal of Public Law*, Vol. XIII (1964), pp. 205–21.
12. Carl Van Doren: *Benjamin Franklin* (New York: The Viking Press; 1938), p. 223.
13. U.S. Senate, Committee on the Judiciary, Subcommittee on Antitrust and Monopoly, 86th Cong., 1st Sess.: *Hearings on Administered Prices* (1959), Pts. 14 and 15; 2nd Sess. (1960), Pts. 16–26.
14. U.S. Senate, Committee on the Judiciary, Subcommittee on Antitrust and Monopoly, 87th Cong., 1st Sess.: *Study of Administered Prices in the Drug Industry* (1961), p. 27.
15. Ibid., pp. 157, 158.
16. U.S. Senate, Committee on the Judiciary, Subcommittee on Antitrust and Monopoly, 87th Cong., 1st and 2nd Sess.: *Hearings on Drug Industry Antitrust Act* (1961, 1962), Pts. 1–7.
17. "The Kefauver Hearings: The Drug Industry Finally Has Its Day and Does Quite Well," *Science*, Vol. CXXXIV (December 15, 1961), pp. 1968–70.
18. H. H. Hussey: "Statement of the American Medical Association Re: S. 1552, 87th Congress Drug Industry Antitrust Act," *The Journal of the American Medical Association*, Vol. CLXXVII (July 22, 1961), pp. 190–5.
19. Raymond Moley: "Kefauver's Inquisition," *Readers' Digest*, December 1961, pp. 69–71.
20. *I. F. Stone's Weekly*, July 17, 1961.
21. "Ethical Drugs—Reflections on the Inquiry," editorial, *New England Journal of Medicine*, Vol. CCLXV (November 16, 1961), pp. 1015–16.
22. "The Kefauver Hearings," loc. cit.
23. Richard Harris: *The Real Voice* (New York: The Macmillan Company; 1964), pp. 171–9.

24. U.S. Senate: *Hearings on Interagency Coordination*, op. cit., Pt. 1, pp. 124–7.
25. *Congressional Record*, Vol. CVIII (August 23, 1962), p. 16,303.
26. Ibid., pp. 16,329, 16,335.
27. Ibid., p. 16,360.
28. U.S. Senate: *Hearings on Interagency Coordination*, op. cit., Pt. 2, pp. 410, 412.
29. Ibid., p. 418.
30. Hubert H. Humphrey: "Myths about Federal Drug Policies," *The New Republic*, May 16, 1964, pp. 10–12.
31. *Congressional Record*, Vol. CIX (April 2, 1963), p. 5115.
32. Stephens Rippey: in U.S. Senate, Committee on Government Operations, Subcommittee on Reorganization and International Organizations, 88th Cong., 1st Sess.: *Hearings on Interagency Coordination in Drug Research and Regulation* (1964), Pt. 4, p. 1823.
33. Ibid., p. 1827.
34. U.S. Senate: *Hearings on Interagency Coordination*, op. cit., Pt. 2, pp. 1186–9.
35. Jonathan Spivak: *The Wall Street Journal*, May 22, 1968, p. 6.
36. Stephens Rippey: *Drug Trade News*, June 17, 1968, p. 45.
37. *Wall Street Journal*, December 11, 1969, p. 2.
38. *FDC Reports*, December 15, 1969, p. 21.
39. *Drug Trade News*, July 29, 1968, p. 7.
40. Roderick Murray: "Biologics Old or New: Research is Vital," *American Professional Pharmacist*, Vol. XXXIII (July 1967), pp. 28–35.
41. U.S. House of Representatives, Committee on Appropriations, Subcommittee, 89th Cong., 2nd Sess.: *Hearings on Department of Health, Education, and Welfare, National Institutes of Health* (1966), Pt. 4, p. 268.
42. Ralph Chester Williams: *The United States Public Health Service 1798–1950* (Washington: Commissioned Officers Association of the U.S. Public Health Service; 1951), pp. 184, 185, 188, 196–198, 209.
43. Roderick Murray: loc. cit., pp. 28–35.
44. U.S. House of Representatives: *Hearings*, op. cit., p. 279.
45. N. Nathanson and A. D. Langmuir: "The Cutter Incident. Polio-

myelitis Following Formaldehyde-Inactivated Poliovirus Vaccination in the United States during the Spring of 1955," *American Journal of Hygiene*, Vol. LXXVIII (July 1963), pp. 16–81, 48, 18–20.

46. Ibid., p. 24.
47. A highly readable summary of these criticisms will be found in John Rowan Wilson: *Margin of Safety* (Garden City, New York: Doubleday and Company, Inc.: 1963), pp. 109–15.
48. Nathanson and Langmuir: loc. cit., p. 24.

CHAPTER 11

1. U.S. Department of Health, Education, and Welfare, Food and Drug Administration, Bureau of Medicine: *Investigational Drug Circular No. 3* (Washington, D.C.; November 2, 1964), p. 1.
2. E. I. Goldenthal: "Current Views on Safety Evaluation of Drugs," *FDA Papers* (May 1968), pp. 13–8.
3. Pharmaceutical Manufacturers Association: "The Investigation of New Drugs: The Conceptual Relation of Studies in Animals to Studies in Man," (Washington, D.C.; 1966).
4. *Congressional Record*, Vol. CVIII (August 23, 1962), p. 16,329.
5. U.S. Senate, Committee on the Judiciary, Subcommittee on Antitrust and Monopoly, 87th Cong., 1st Sess.: *Hearings on Drug Industry Antitrust Act* (1961), Pt. 1, p. 59.
6. 21 Code of Federal Regulations, Section 130.37 (1968).
7. Ibid.
8. U.S. Senate, Committee on Government Operations, Subcommittee on Reorganization and International Organizations, 88th Cong., 1st Sess.: *Hearings on Interagency Coordination in Drug Research and Regulation* (1964), Pt. 4, pp. 1652–9.
9. Letter from William H. Stewart, Surgeon General, U.S. Public Health Service, to heads of institutions conducting research with Public Health Service grants, February 8, 1966.
10. U.S. Senate: *Hearings on Drug Industry Antitrust Act*, op. cit., p. 417.
11. U.S. Senate, Select Committee on Small Business, Subcommittee

on Monopoly, 90th Cong., 1st Sess.: *Hearings on Competitive Problems in the Drug Industry* (1967), Pt. 1, pp. 258–281.

12. "FDA Orders Clinical Tests of Generic," *Medical World News*, Vol. IX (January 5, 1968), p. 23.

13. *Drug Research Reports*, Vol. X No. 52 (December 27, 1967).

14. R. M. Hodges: "Biopharmaceutic Equivalency and the Role of the Food and Drug Administration," *American Journal of Hospital Pharmacy*, Vol. XXV (March 1968), pp. 121–7.

15. *Drug Trade News*, May 20, 1968.

16. U.S. Department of Health, Education, and Welfare, Office of the Secretary: *Task Force on Prescription Drugs: Final Report* (Washington, D.C.; February 7, 1969), p. 34.

17. Herbert L. Ley, Jr.: "Problems of the Investigational Drug Regulations," *Chicago Medicine*, Vol. LXX (June 24, 1967), pp. 493–7.

18. U.S. Senate, Committee on Government Operations, Subcommittee on Reorganization and International Organizations, 88th Cong., 1st Sess.: *Hearings on Interagency Coordination in Drug Research and Regulation* (1964), Pt. 4, p. 1678.

19. Paul de Haen: "Drugs and Drug Use," *Medical Science*, Vol. XVIII (June 1967), pp. 12–16, 58–64.

20. Herbert L. Ley, Jr.: "FDA Today and Tomorrow." Paper presented at the 12th Food, Drug and Law Institute, Food and Drug Administration, Joint Educational Conference (Washington D.C.; December 3, 1968).

21. R. M. Hodges: "The Review and Processing of New Drug Applications," *FDA Papers* (July–August 1967), pp. 27–30.

22. Jonathan Will: "The Feminine Conscience of FDA: Dr. Frances Oldham Kelsey," *Saturday Review*, September 1, 1962, pp. 41–3.

23. U.S. Senate: *Hearings on Interagency Coordination*, op. cit., Pt. 6, p. 3020.

24. A. B. Sabin: "Amantadine Hydrochloride: Analysis of Data Related to Its Proposed Use for Prevention of A2 Influenza Virus Disease in Human Beings," *The Journal of the American Medical Association*, Vol. CC (June 12, 1967), pp. 135–42.

25. U.S. Senate: *Hearings on Interagency Coordination*, op. cit. (1963), Pt. 3, pp. 984–5.

26. Ibid. (1964), Pt. 6, pp. 3004–6.

27. U.S. Senate, Committee on Government Operations, Subcommittee on Reorganization and International Organizations, 89th Cong., 2nd Sess.: *Interagency Drug Coordination* (1966), p. 40.
28. Ibid., pp. 42–3.
29. Letter to the author from Charlotte Gallogly, Bureau of Medicine, FDA, January 11, 1968.
30. *Drug Research Reports*, Vol. XI (July 10, 1968), p. 4.
31. W. H. Summerson: "The Role of Scientific Research in the Food and Drug Administration," *Food, Drug and Cosmetic Law Journal*, Vol. XX (July 1965), pp. 427–32.
32. L. T. Coggeshall: "The University and the Food and Drug Administration," *Clinical Research*, Vol. XII (October 1964), pp. 311–14.
33. *Drug Research Reports*, Vol. XI (June 26, 1968), pp. 10–13.
34. Oscar E. Anderson, Jr.: *The Health of a Nation, Harvey W. Wiley and the Fight for Pure Food* (Chicago: University of Chicago Press; 1958), pp. 106–13.
35. U.S. Senate: *Hearings on Interagency Coordination*, op. cit. (1963), Pt. 3, p. 1040.
36. W. W. Wright and A. Kirshbaum: "National Center for Antibiotics and Insulin Analysis," *FDA Papers* (May 1968), pp. 23–4.
37. U.S. Department of Health, Education, and Welfare, Office of the Secretary: *National Academy of Sciences—National Research Council, Report of Special Committee to Secretary of Health, Education, and Welfare to Review the Policies, Procedures, and Decisions of the Division of Antibiotics and the New Drug Branch of the Food and Drug Administration*, October 6, 1960.
38. Wright and Kirshbaum: loc. cit.
39. U.S. Department of Health, Education, and Welfare: *1968 Annual Report* (Washington, D.C.: Government Printing Office; 1969), p. 332.
40. F. J. Ayd: "Should All Drugs Be Available for Use by All Physicians?" *Medical Science*, Vol. XVIII (December 1967), pp. 35–42.
41. Letter to the author from John J. Jennings, Bureau of Medicine, FDA, August 14, 1968.
42. *Drug Research Reports*, Vol. XI (July 10, 1968), p. 4.
43. 76 Stat. 788–9.

44. "The Washington Briefing on FDA's Drug Efficacy Review, Question and Answer Session," *FDA Papers* (March 1968), pp. 19, 29–31.
45. 33 Fed. Reg. 818 (1968).
46. "At the Editor's Desk," *Illinois Medical Journal*, Vol. CXI (January 1957), pp. 52–3.
47. *Drug Trade News*, May 5, 1969, p. 1.
48. W. H. W. Inman and M. P. Vessey: "Investigation of Deaths from Pulmonary, Coronary, and Cerebral Thrombosis and Embolism in Women of Child-Bearing Age," *British Medical Journal*, Vol. II (April 27, 1968), pp. 193–9; M. P. Vessey and R. Doll: "Investigation of Relation Between Use of Oral Contraceptives and Thromboembolic Disease," *British Medical Journal*, Vol. II (April 27, 1968), pp. 199–205.
49. J. F. Sadusk and P. A. Palmisano: "Teratogenic Effect of Meclizine, Cyclizine and Chlorcyclizine," *The Journal of the American Medical Association*, Vol. CXCIV (November 29, 1965), pp. 987–9.
50. N. L. Chayet: "Power of the Package Insert," *New England Journal of Medicine*, Vol. CCLXXVII (December 7, 1967), pp. 1253–4.
51. "The FDA Under Dr. Ley," *Medical World News*, Vol. IX, (August 16, 1968), pp. 14–16.
52. Walter Modell: "FDA Censorship," editorial, *Clinical Pharmacology and Therapeutics*, Vol. VIII (May–June 1967), pp. 359–61.
53. Herbert L. Ley, Jr.: "FDA Papers (Letter to the Editor)," *Clinical Pharmacology and Therapeutics*, Vol. VIII (September–October 1967), pp. 749–51.
54. Julius Hauser: "Medical Communications: Law, Ethics and Booby Traps," *Clinical Pharmacology and Therapeutics*, Vol. IX (March–April 1968), pp. 271–6.
55. U.S. Department of Health, Education, and Welfare, Office of the Secretary: *Task Force on Prescription Drugs, Second Interim Report and Recommendations* (Washington, D.C.; August 30, 1968), p. 71.
56. "Summary: President Johnson's Health Message," *The Journal of the American Medical Association*, Vol. CCIII (March 25, 1968), pp. 41–2.

57. "FDA's Compendium: Easier Idea: Easier Said Than Done," editorial, *Drug Trade News*, July 31, 1967, p. 20.
58. U.S. Department of Health, Education, and Welfare, Food and Drug Administration: *Compendium of Medical Advertising, FDA Publication No. 40* (Washington, D.C.: Government Printing Office; June 1967), pp. 5–6.
59. Ibid., pp. 2–4.
60. "Medical Advertising: State of the Craft and of Regulation," *FDA Papers* (February 1967), pp. 4–8.
61. U.S. Department of Health, Education and Welfare: *Compendium*, op. cit., p. 26.
62. *Drug Trade News*, November 21, 1966, p. 1.
63. U.S. Senate, Select Committee on Small Business, Subcommittee on Monopoly, United States Senate, 90th Cong., 2nd Sess., 91st Cong., 1st Sess.: *Hearings on Competitive Problems in the Drug Industry* (1969), Pt. 10, p. 4115.
64. "Medical Advertising," loc. cit., p. 7.
65. 34 Fed. Reg. 7802 (1969).
66. *Drug Trade News*, August 12, 1968, p. 2.
67. E. S. Turner: *The Shocking History of Advertising!* (New York: E. P. Dutton & Co., Inc.; 1953), p. 169.
68. U.S. Senate: *Interagency Drug Coordination*, op. cit., pp. 18–19.
69. James L. Goddard: "Shared Responsibilities," in *Compendium of Medical Advertising, FDA Publication No. 40* (Washington, D.C.: Government Printing Office; June 1967), pp. 24–7.
70. Jonathan Spivak: "Goddard, Quitting FDA, Takes With Him High Public Reputation, Unfulfilled Goals," *Wall Street Journal*, May 22, 1966, p. 6.
71. U.S. House of Representatives, Committee on Government Operations, Subcommittee, 88th Cong., 2nd Sess.: *Hearings on Drug Safety* (1964), Pt. 1, p. 217.
72. Vincent A. Kleinfeld: "New Drug Applications and Suspension Procedures," *Food, Drug and Cosmetic Law Journal*, Vol. XVIII (November 1963), pp. 632–41.
73. D. F. Cavers: "Administering That Ounce of Prevention: New Drugs and Nuclear Reactors—I," *West Virginia Law Review*, Vol. LXVIII (February 1966), pp. 109–35.
74. "Abbott Labs Acquitted on PDR Case," *Hospital Tribune*, August 12, 1968, p. 3.

75. Kleinfeld: loc. cit.
76. W. C. Warren: "Congressional Investigations: Some Observations," *Food, Drug and Cosmetic Law Journal,* Vol. XXI (1966), pp. 40, 45, cited in D. F. Cavers: "Administering That Ounce of Prevention: New Drugs and Nuclear Reactors—II," *West Virginia Law Review,* Vol. LXVIII (April 1966), pp. 233–62.
77. Cavers: ibid., p. 259.
78. D. C. Hansen: "Illinois' New Food and Drug Act," *FDA Papers,* Vol. II (March 1968), pp. 4–6.
79. Cited in Elizabeth B. Drew: "Is the FCC Dead?" *Atlantic Monthly,* July 1967, pp. 29–36.
80. Alfred North Whitehead: *The Aims of Education and Other Essays* (New York: New American Library of World Literature, Inc.; 1954), p. 26.
81. U.S. House of Representatives: *Hearings on Drug Safety,* op. cit., pp. 156–8.
82. Austin Smith and Arthur D. Herrick, eds.: *Drug Research and Development* (New York: Revere Publishing Co.; 1948), p. 5.
83. J. Bronowski: *Science and Human Values* (New York: Julian Messner, Inc.; 1956), p. 81.
84. E. P. Herring: *Public Administration and the Public Interest,* 1967 ed. (New York: Russell and Russell; 1936), p. 16.

CHAPTER 12

1. *Pharmacopoeia Londinensis of 1681. Reproduced in Facsimile,* with a Historical Introduction by George Urdang (Madison, Wisconsin: State Historical Society of Wisconsin; 1944).
2. A. C. Corcoran, ed.: *A Mirror Up to Medicine* (Philadelphia: J. B. Lippincott Co.; 1961), p. 112.
3. S. T. Anning: "A Hospital Pharmacopoeia of the Nineteenth Century," *Medical History,* Vol. X (January 1966), pp. 70–5.
4. G. W. Jones: "Robert Boyle as a Medical Man," *Bulletin of the History of Medicine,* Vol. XXXVIII (March–April 1964), pp. 139–52.
5. H. C. Wood, cited in Alex Berman: "The Heroic Approach in

19th Century Therapeutics," *University of Michigan Medical Bulletin*, Vol. XXIV (November 1958), pp. 419–27. This article gives an excellent review of the practices of this period.

6. John Forbes, cited in Berman, ibid., p. 424.

7. William Osler: *The Principles and Practice of Medicine*, 1st ed. (New York: D. Appleton and Company; 1892), pp. 253, 529, 716.

8. U.S. Department of Health, Education, and Welfare: *Task Force on Prescription Drugs. Background Papers. The Drug Users*, advance ed. (Washington, D.C.; October 1, 1968), pp. 26, 43.

9. "Report of the First Teaching Institute, Association of American Medical Colleges. The Teaching of Physiology, Biochemistry, Pharmacology," *Journal of Medical Education*, Vol. XXIX (July 1954), Pt. 2, p. 113.

10. George W. Corner: *Two Centuries of Medicine. A History of the School of Medicine of the University of Pennsylvania* (Philadelphia: J. B. Lippincott Company; 1965), p. 81.

11. James S. Coleman, Elihu Katz and Herbert Menzel: *Medical Innovation. A Diffusion Study* (Indianapolis: The Bobbs-Merrill Company, Inc.; 1966), p. 59.

12. R. Ferber and H. G. Wales: "The Effectiveness of Pharmaceutical Promotion," *University of Illinois Bureau of Economics and Business Research Bulletin 83* (Urbana, Illinois; 1958), p. 24.

13. *Attitudes of U. S. Physicians Toward the American Pharmaceutical Industry* (Chicago: Ben Gaffin and Associates, Inc.; 1959), p. C-13.

14. Ibid., p. C-16.

15. Pharmaceutical Manufacturers Association: "Survey of Physicians" (Washington, D.C.; 1960), quoted in J. J. Harris: "Survey of Medical Communication. Sources Available for Continuing Physician Education," *Journal of Medical Education*, Vol. XLI (August 1966), pp. 737–55.

16. *Report of the Committee of Enquiry into the Relationship of the Pharmaceutical Industry with the National Health Service 1965–67* (London: Her Majesty's Stationery Office; 1967), pp. 137–8.

17. Ibid., p. 143.

18. Ibid., p. 151.

19. Coleman and others, op. cit., pp. 133–8.
20. Harry F. Dowling and others: "Pneumococcal Meningitis. A Study of Seventy-Two Cases," *New England Journal of Medicine*, Vol. CCXXVI (June 25, 1942), pp. 1015–18.
21. M. D. Sheps and A. P. Shapiro: "The Physician's Responsibility in the Age of Therapeutic Plenty," *Circulation*, Vol. XXV (February 1962), pp. 399–407; U.S. Department of Health, Education, and Welfare, Public Health Service, National Center for Health Statistics: *Vital Statistics of the United States* (Washington, D.C.: Government Printing Office), Vol. II, 1959, p. 35; Vol. II, Part A, 1960, p. 34; 1961, p. 34; 1962, p. 71; 1963, p. 70; 1964, p. 85; 1965, p. 85.
22. C. Muller: "Medical Review of Prescribing," *Journal of Chronic Diseases*, Vol. XVIII (July 1965), pp. 689–96.
23. U.S. Senate, Committee on Government Operations, Subcommittee on Reorganization and International Organizations, 88th Cong., 1st Sess.: *Hearings on Interagency Coordination in Drug Research and Regulation* (1964), Pt. 6, pp. 3146–9.
24. R. S. Myers: "The Misuse of Antibacterials in Inguinal Herniorrhaphy," *Surgery, Gynecology and Obstetrics*, Vol. CVIII (June 1959), pp. 721–5.
25. C. N. Lewis and others: "Chloramphenicol (Chloromycetin) in Relation to Blood Dyscrasias with Observations in Other Drugs," *Antibiotics and Chemotherapy*, Vol. II (December 1952), pp. 601–9.
26. W. Dameshek: "Chloramphenicol—A New Warning," *The Journal of the American Medical Association*, Vol. 174 (December 3, 1960), pp. 1853–4.
27. U.S. Senate, Select Committee on Small Business, Subcommittee on Monopoly, 90th Cong., 2nd Sess.: *Hearings on Competitive Problems in the Drug Industry* (1968), Pt. 9, p. 3554.
28. W. R. Best: "Chloramphenicol-Associated Blood Dyscrasias," *The Journal of the American Medical Association*, Vol. CCI (July 17, 1967), pp. 181–8.
29. U.S. Senate: *Hearings on Competitive Problems in the Drug Industry*, op. cit., 1st and 2nd Sess. (1968), Pt. 6, p. 2639.
30. D. W. Richards: "A Clinician's View of Advances in Therapeutics," in Paul Talalay, ed.: *Drugs in Our Society* (Baltimore: The Johns Hopkins Press; 1964), p. 33.

31. E. Freidson: "Client Control of Medical Practice," *American Journal of Sociology*, Vol. LXV (January 1960), pp. 374–82.
32. S. Crosbie and H. Gilberstadt: "Contrasts Between Several Means of Appraising Physicians," *Journal of Medical Education*, Vol. XXXVI (October 1961), pp. 1310–5.
33. C. Smith: "How Good is Your Family Doctor?" *Atlantic Monthly*, August 1950, pp. 43–7.
34. O. L. Peterson and others: "An Analytical Study of North Carolina General Practice, 1953–1954," *Journal of Medical Education*, Vol. XXXI (December 1956), Pt. 2, pp. 121, 39–43, 19.
35. Kenneth F. Clute: *The General Practitioner. A Study of Medical Education and Practice in Ontario and Nova Scotia* (Toronto: University of Toronto Press; 1963), pp. 300–1.

CHAPTER 13

1. G. H. Brieger: "Therapeutic Conflicts and the American Medical Profession in the 1860's," *Bulletin of the History of Medicine*, Vol. XLI (May–June 1967), pp. 215–22.
2. Harry F. Dowling: "How Do Practicing Physicians Use New Drugs?" *The Journal of the American Medical Association*, Vol. CLXXXV (July 27, 1963), pp. 233–6.
3. James Howard Means: *The Association of American Physicians. Its First Seventy-Five Years* (New York: McGraw-Hill Book Company, Inc.; 1961).
4. Bernhard J. Stern: *Society and Medical Progress* (Princeton, New Jersey: Princeton University Press; 1941), pp. 175–214.
5. Michael F. C. Crick: *Adverse Drug Reactions* (Cambridge, Mass.: Bolt, Beranek and Newman Incorporated; March, 1968), Report No. 1582.
6. Ibid., pp. 31–2.
7. E. A. Carr, Jr.: "Proposed Aims, Organization, and Activities of a Division of Clinical Pharmacology," *Clinical Pharmacology and Therapeutics*, Vol. IV (September–October 1963), pp. 587–95.
8. S. Garb: "The Reaction of Medical Students to Drug Advertising," *New England Journal of Medicine*, Vol. CCLIX (July 17, 1958), pp. 121–3.
9. C. H. Ward and K. Rickels: "The Double-Blind Drug Study as

a Teaching Device," *Journal of Medical Education*, Vol. XXXVI (May 1961), pp. 410–13.

10. R. F. Palmer: "Drug Misuse and Physician Education," *Clinical Pharmacology and Therapeutics*, Vol. X (January–February 1969), pp. 1–4.

11. Osler L. Peterson and others: "An Analytical Study of North Carolina General Practice, 1953–1954," *Journal of Medical Education*, Vol. XXXI (December 1956), Pt. 2, p. 65.

12. Ibid., pp. 76, 80.

13. Council on Medical Education, American Medical Association: "Medical Education in the United States. Section IV: Continuing Medical Education," *The Journal of the American Medical Association*, Vol. CCVI (November 25, 1968), pp. 2048–53.

14. C. H. W. Ruhe, R. W. Howard, and E. Roughley: "Continuing Education for Physicians for the Period from September 1, 1968 to August 31, 1969," *The Journal of the American Medical Association*, Vol. CCV (August 5, 1968), pp. 353–458.

15. S. Abrahamson: "Evaluation in Continuing Medical Education," *The Journal of the American Medical Association*, Vol. CCVI (October 14, 1968), pp. 625–8. This is an excellent discussion of the objectives and methods of evaluation.

16. Douglas D. Vollan: *Postgraduate Medical Education in the United States* (Chicago: American Medical Association; 1955), p. 47.

17. C. H. Castle and P. B. Storey: "Physicians' Needs and Interests in Continuing Medical Education," *The Journal of the American Medical Association*, Vol. CCVI (October 14, 1968), pp. 611–14.

18. *Joint Commission on Accreditation of Hospitals, Bulletin No. 40* (Chicago; December, 1965), pp. 2–3.

19. U.S. Senate, Select Committee on Small Business, Subcommittee on Monopoly, 90th Cong., 1st and 2nd Sess.: *Hearings on Competitive Problems in the Drug Industry* (1968), Pt. 6, p. 2617.

20. D. F. Burkholder: "Drugs Selected by Pharmacy and Therapeutic Committees of Teaching Hospitals," *Drug Intelligence*, Vol. I (October 1967), pp. 321–9.

21. C. Muller and R. Westheimer: "Formularies and Drug Standards in Metropolitan Hospitals," *Hospitals*, Vol. XL (January 16, 1966).

22. U.S. Senate: *Hearings on Competitive Problems*, op. cit., 1st Sess. (1967), Pt. 2, p. 589.

23. "M.D. Self-Policing Uses Blue Shield Data," *Medical World News*, March 15, 1968, pp. 28–9.
24. Vollan: op. cit., p. 50.
25. Ibid.
26. "Where M.D.'s Must Keep Up or Get Out," *Medical World News*, July 5, 1968, pp. 14–15.
27. William Osler: *Aphorisms from His Bedside Teachings and Writings*, William B. Bean, ed. (Springfield, Illinois: Charles C. Thomas; 1961), p. 54.
28. C. N. Mohler, D. G. Wallin, and E. G. Dreyfus: "Studies in the Home Treatment of Streptococcal Disease. I. Failure of Patients to Take Penicillin by Mouth as Prescribed," *New England Journal of Medicine*, Vol. CCLII (June 30, 1955), pp. 1116–18.
29. A. B. Bergman and R. J. Werner: "Failure of Children to Receive Penicillin by Mouth," *New England Journal of Medicine*, Vol. CCLXVIII (June 13, 1963), pp. 1334–8.
30. D. R. C. Willcox, R. Gillan, and E. H. Hare: "Do Psychiatric Out-Patients Take Their Drugs," *British Medical Journal*, Vol. II (October 2, 1965), pp. 790–2.
31. Herbert S. Caron and Harold P. Roth: "Patients' Cooperation with a Medical Regimen: Difficulties in Identifying the Non-cooperator," *The Journal of the American Medical Association*, Vol. CCIII (March 11, 1968), pp. 922–6.
32. Francis Weld Peabody: "The Care of the Patient," in *Doctor and Patient. Papers on the Relationship of the Physician to Men and Institutions* (New York: The Macmillan Company; 1930), p. 57.

CHAPTER 14

1. George S. Shakespeare, Jr.: "The Moral Imperatives of Television," in Fulton J. Quinn, ed.: *Ethics, Advertising and Responsibility* (Westminster, Maryland: Canterbury Press; 1963), pp. 77–81.

Index

Abbott Laboratories, 41, 256
Accepted Dental Remedies (American Dental Association), 184–5
acetanilide, 190
administered prices, 109, 133
advertising, 121–35, 272–4, 286–7, 291, 304; effect of, on doctors, 116, 123, 124–5, 197–8; expenditures for, 122–123; volume of, 122–3; misleading, 124–6; medical students and, 124, 125; Food and Drug Administration (FDA) and, 250–4; *see also* detail men
Agriculture, Department of, 35, 43
Alabama Medical Society, 64
Aldomet, 252
alkaloids, 16
Alsberg, Carl L., 191
Altafur, 256
amantadine, 22, 226
American Academy of General Practice, 294, 303
American Academy of Pediatrics, 74
American College of Physicians, 296, 298
American College of Surgeons, 298
American Cyanamid Company, 84, 85, 89

American Dental Association: Council on Dental Therapeutics of, 139, 174, 184–5; Seal of Acceptance Program of, 184–5; advertising of drugs and, 185
American Home Products Corporation, 84
American Hospital Association, 298
American Hospital Formulary Service, 270, 290
American Medical Association (AMA), 153–84; Council on Drugs of, 147, 162–6, 177–9, 182–3, 184, 221, 235, 248; Council on Pharmacy and Chemistry of, 39, 147, 154–162, 166, 169, 170, 172, 173, 175, 177, 180, 184, 189; names of drugs and, 144–5, 166–7, 182–3; *Epitome of the United States Pharmacopeia and the National Formulary*, publication of, 147, 176; advertising of drugs and, 154–155, 160–2, 169, 171–3, 179, 180–1; Seal of Acceptance Program of, 154, 160, 162, 166, 171–7, 180, 184; Council on Medical Education of, 155, 182; Council on Foods and Nutrition of, 160; Council on Physical Medicine of, 160;

A NOTE ABOUT THE AUTHOR

Dr. Harry F. Dowling was born in Washington, D.C., in 1904. He received his B.A. degree (magna cum laude) *from Franklin and Marshall College, his M.D. degree (with distinction) from The George Washington University School of Medicine, and completed his residency training at Johns Hopkins University and Harvard University. Affiliated with The George Washington University School of Medicine, he ultimately served as Clinical Professor of Medicine and Chief of the university's division at Gallinger Municipal Hospital. In 1950 he joined the faculty of the University of Illinois College of Medicine and in 1951 assumed duties as the head of their department of Internal Medicine. In 1969 he became Professor Emeritus and is now associated with the University of Delaware as Special Assistant to the President for Medical Affairs.*

Dr. Dowling's primary field of research has been infectious diseases, including the methods of action of serums, sulfonamides, and antibiotics. He is the author of more than two hundred scientific articles and several books. Active in the field of drug therapy, Dr. Dowling has served on the Revision Committee of the U.S. Pharmacopeia *since 1956, the AMA Council on Drugs (1960–6, Chairman 1963–6), and the Medical Advisory Board of the FDA since 1965. He is a member of many medical associations and is a Fellow of the American College of Physicians and a Diplomate of the American Board of Internal Medicine. Dr. Dowling is married and is the father of three grown sons.*

A NOTE ON THE TYPE

The text of this book is set in Caledonia, *a
Linotype face designed by W. A. Dwiggins. It
belongs to the family of printing types called
"modern face" by printers—a term used to mark
the change in style of type-letters that occurred
about 1800. Caledonia borders on the general
design of Scotch Modern, but is more freely drawn
than that letter.*

*The book was composed, printed, and bound by
The Haddon Craftsmen, Scranton, Pennsylvania.*